EMPOWERED

EMPOWERED

*Essential Concepts and Strategies
Every Woman Should Know About
Self Defense*

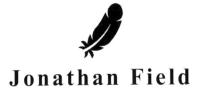

Jonathan Field

Dedication

This book is dedicated to the strong and dedicated women I have had the distinct pleasure to teach, work, and train with.

You are an inspiration to all the women out there who need someone to look up to.

TABLE OF CONTENT

FOREWORD

O n average a woman is killed in Canada every two days. Once a week a woman is murdered by her partner and one in three women will experience some sort of sexual violence during their lifetime. Yet, studies show only 1% of women actually report these incidents. While reading this I ask myself, what is wrong with society to allow these statistics? Why is there not more focus on women's violence? What can be done?

As many parents would agree, especially those of little girls, the moment your baby enters the world fears that you would have never put a second thought to become amplified. The above statistics become very real. How can we as parents equip our young girls to handle these unthinkable realities?

Knowledge is power! This book is the first step in that process. We are all worth defending and you have the strength to do it. Through this reading, Master Jonathan Field will take you on a journey of awareness and self-empowerment. He will describe basic yet potentially lifesaving defense techniques that we are all capable of mastering as well as real life stories of situations women sadly encounter. He will guide you into furthering that knowledge mentally and physically. You will feel empowered!

My journey began with Cobourg Tae Kwon Do many years ago. I had taken time to settle down and start my family and decided it was time to invest time in myself. I dabbled in some martial arts as a teenager and knew exactly what I was looking for. I wanted a martial arts workout minus the combativeness of martial arts classes. To my luck, I found Cobourg Tae Kwon Do which offered a Fitness Kickboxing class. It was exactly what I was looking for. Workouts were similar to that of MMA style training. There were actual heavy bags to kick, and focus mitts to punch. I could feel what it was like to actually hit something and condition myself to that. I was able to rebuild strength and learn simple techniques to defend myself. With strength and confidence building, I had decided to take the next step, face my fears and join Taekwondo. I am now a 2nd Degree Black Belt.

As a mother of three young girls and advocate for women's empowerment, I encourage women of all ages to read this book. Violence against women is often a silent war. We must equip ourselves and our children with the tools to defend, and knowledge to recognize dangerous situations. We must choose to empower ourselves, build confidence and reflect that on others. Together we can break this silence!

You have the right to defend yourself and
you are worth defending!

Cheryl Sanders

INTRODUCTION

I started my Taekwondo and Martial Arts career back on February 11, 1998. That was the day my father signed me up for Taekwondo lessons at Cobourg Tae Kwon Do. A Taekwondo academy I would purchase from my first Taekwondo instructor five short years later while studying Business Administration and Supervisory Management in college. I was one of those students that would go to classes pretty much every day. I was obsessed with learning Martial Arts. All areas including forms, self-defense, weapons, sparring, breaking, and the many other aspects of the arts.

Many years later, after winning multiple championships, including World Championships in both the International Sports Karate Association and the World Breaking Association, I became interested in teaching self-defense seminars to women. I would teach the odd workshop for women's groups, local businesses, or parents who hired me to teach their daughters. Working with hundreds of girls and women at the academy and producing some world champions and quality female black belts, I became increasingly interested in expanding our self-defense seminars.

The seminars had to be more than just physical techniques or the traditional 'when this happens; you do this' experience. Attendees needed to learn about how ninety percent of self-defense is mental, and ten percent is the physical, which we try to avoid at all costs. Another thing that had to change was keeping the defense techniques extremely simple so that anyone could make them work regardless of size or strength. Plus, the seminars had to focus on empowering women.

After teaching a few self-defense seminars with one of my female Black Belts, Cheryl, the concepts of Women's Empowerment and Defense Workshops was born. Our empowerment workshops continue to evolve each time we conduct one as new information and experiences cross our paths. During each one of our workshops, the attendees receive a free copy of our Women's Empowerment and Defense Guide. From this came the idea to write this book as I feel every woman needs to know the concepts and strategies within these pages.

After spending nearly twenty years of working with women at the academy and at the various workshops, and such, I have seen the aftermaths of sexual assaults and abuse. The abuse or assault isn't just a one-time thing and you get over it. No, I see women suffering ten, twenty, thirty, and more years after. The trauma of the incidents, stick with them on a daily basis. Sometimes it is just as real today as it was when it first happened. One of the goals of this book is to help reduce the number of assaults and abuse that happen to women.

How you should use this book is to read it through cover-to-cover. Enjoy the main story of Miesha located between each section, as well as the various other stories and examples within these pages. Afterward, go through the book a few more initial times and implement the empowerment and defense concepts and strategies into your daily lives. Then every so often, perhaps once every few months, skim through the pages to remind yourself of the main points to help keep the concepts and strategies in this book fresh in your mind.

Empowered: Essential Concepts and Strategies Every Woman Should Know About Self-Defense is divided into ten main chapters. Each chapter will cover one aspect of self-protection and empowerment. Within any given part, there will be multiple concepts, strategies, ideas, and stories relating to that section. Some of the concepts and strategies can and will overlap each other, and no single self-protection concept can stand-alone. That being said, some concepts can apply to multiple aspects of self-defense; however, I put them in this book where I feel they fit best.

CHAPTER ONE
LET'S START WITH YOU

So this book is primarily about learning and practicing the ninety percent of self-protection, which is the mental aspect. The more you focus on the psychological aspects and strategies to keep yourself safe, the less likely you will have to use the remaining ten percent, which is your physical game. That should be your goal, to avoid having to use the physical side of self-protection to defend yourself from a dangerous situation or attacker.

To accomplish this, we must first take a look at you. Because most of the time, it is you who is responsible for keeping you out of harm's way. Now I am not saying it is your fault if someone decides to attack or harm you. Not at all, rather that you must be proactive in staying alert and take responsibility for your safety. Sometimes bad people will do horrible things to others, and it's unavoidable. But you can reduce the risk by implementing self-protection strategies in your day-to-day routines.

Your Right To Fight Back

First of all, let's start by stating that you have every right to fight back and defend yourself. Reread this; you have every right to fight back and protect yourself. No one has the right to abuse you in any way, whether that be physical, mental, emotional, or verbal.

Whether the attack from your assailant is physical or verbal, you need to stand up for yourself. Statistics show that women who stand up or fight back are less likely to sustain serious injuries or worse from their assailants. Most attackers do not attack potential victims if they believe they will fight back.

You have the right to fight back, so exercise this right. Obviously, I am talking about the scenarios where self-defense is genuinely needed and not just a minor disagreement or conflict with someone else. Defending yourself with physicality should only occur if there is a reasonable assumption that someone is going to hurt you physically, and you cannot leave the situation safely.

Now when it comes to verbal altercations, you have to gauge the situation a little more carefully. If you are arguing with someone, you can't just go ahead and hit them. However, if you are in a situation where you feel that things have escalated to the point that you fear you will be hurt if you don't defend yourself first, you may act first.

Many factors play into scenarios where you pre-emptive strike. Meaning you can strike first without your assailant initiating the physicality. Factors such as the composure of the attacker, are you trapped somewhere where you can't escape, the words they are using, their physical size and strength compared to yours, and their intention towards you.

Know Your Worth

You need to understand that you are extremely important in this world. You have friends who love you. If you are lucky enough to have both your parents, they love you. If you are married with children or married without children, they all love you. Or perhaps you have that special someone that makes you smile every time you think about them; they love you too. Even any pets that you have love you. Regardless of the combination of people above, you are loved.

But to you, all this may not matter if you don't love yourself and see your self-worth. You need to realize that you are a unique person who contributes to many lives. Merely being you, you make other people's lives better. You have talents and skills that are unique to you. You add value to this world. Take a few moments each day to appreciate yourself for who you are, what you have (not just material-wise), and what you have accomplished so far.

You owe it to yourself and to those who love you to keep yourself safe from potentially dangerous situations that are mostly avoidable through daily active practices of self-defense. You do not want to find yourself on the wrong end of a situation that could be avoided by practicing good self-defense habits daily.

Know Your Strengths

Everyone, including you, has natural strengths. Things you are good at naturally and skills you have spent the time to learn. It is no different when it comes to self-defense. There will be skills, techniques, and concepts that you will naturally be good at without much effort. Then there will be those skills and concepts you will have to work at to become effective at executing.

You will need to figure out what your strengths are and what your weaknesses are—both in the mental and physical games. Let's first take a look at your mental game. As you read through this book and learn about all the various concepts and strategies, take notes on the things you are already doing well. Then think about how you can make yourself better at the strategies you are good at and how you can improve upon them to make it work better for you.

Now you need to take notes on the concepts you are not as good at or maybe even not doing at all. Most likely, there will be strategies and ideas in here you have never thought about before. That is okay. They, unfortunately, don't teach a lot of this in school. Most likely, you may not even have had conversations with other people about self-defense and empowerment.

Once you have notes on all the things you are not doing, decide to implement strategies into your daily practice. You don't have to do them all at once. There's too many of them for that, and you'll forget. Best practice is to start by adding one that you feel is best suited for your daily life and needs. After a week or so when you feel you are getting pretty good at this new skill, add another one. Keep repeating the process one skill at a time until you have many self-defense tools in your toolbox.

Now, as the main focus of this book is to teach you about the mental aspects of keeping yourself safe and out of harm's way, we will cover a bit about the physical side of self-defense right here. It is essential to know your physical strengths against an assailant. The human body is a fantastic machine of biomechanical strengths and weaknesses. We will cover weaknesses later on in a different section, so let's explore your physical strengths.

Nature has given you a bunch of physical tools that you can use to defend yourself in physical altercations. Regardless of your size or perceived strengths or weaknesses, these techniques are powerful.

Hand And Arm Strikes

- Palm Strikes
- Punches
- Hammer Fists
- Slaps
- Finger and Thumb Pokes

- Elbow Strikes
- Ridge Hand Strikes
- Knife Hand Strikes

Kicks and Knee Strikes

- Heel Stomp
- Roundhouse Kick
- Side Kick
- Back Kick
- Front Kick
- Snap Kick
- Knee Strike

There are a few key points to know about these self-protection strikes. First, use soft surface techniques such as palm strikes, slaps, and hammer fists on hard surfaces such as the face and skull. You are less likely to injure yourself. Second, elbows are effective strikes no matter where they hit. Third, strikes like punches, ridge hands, and knife hand strikes are better for striking soft targets like the ribs, solar plexus, kidneys, neck, throat, and groin. Again, you are less likely to injure yourself yet cause a lot of pain and damage to your assailant. Fourth, finger and thumb pokes are effective against the eyes and throat—extremely vulnerable parts of your body.

As powerful as the hand and arm strikes can be, your legs are more powerful. Just compare the sheer size and power of the legs to your arms, and you will realize where your strengths lie. Here are a few quick points for kicking. One, heel stomps cause a lot of pain and damage on the top of your assailant's feet. Two, roundhouse kicks, sidekicks, back kicks, and front kicks to the knees will cause a lot of damage and will put your attacker down. Three, knee strikes are brutal against the body, head, and groin. Four, kicks can be used on your assailant to cause pain and damage, create space between you and them so you can escape, or put them down for the count.

The above is just a brief overview of the basic combative strikes used in self-protection. You will learn a bit more in the section that covers your assailant's weaknesses later in the book. For more details on various self-defense techniques and the scenarios you would use, check out the companion to this book coming out soon (depending when you are reading this book), *Physical Empowerment: Essential Self-Defense Techniques Every Woman Should Know About Self-Defense.*

Trust Your Intuitions

Have you ever had that feeling in your gut that told you something is not quite right? The answer is probably yes, we all have. That gut feeling, or some describe it as butterflies in your stomach, or perhaps your spidey sense is tingling. That's nature's way of letting you know something is wrong. Often people will ignore these feelings for various reasons which can put their lives in danger.

Such reasons can include not wanting to offend someone, thinking they are just being silly, or nothing bad will happen to me. These reasons can get you in a lot of trouble. What you should do is listen to your intuition and assess the current circumstance to figure out what is causing you to have such feelings. Once you know what is causing the gut reaction, you can make a smart decision to do the things that will keep you safe. Let's take a look at Hazel.

Hazel was getting off work quite late on a Friday night. She was looking forward to spending the weekend hanging out with her friends. They were going to start the weekend that night at one of the local pubs. But first she was heading to her bank to get some cash out of the ATM so she wouldn't have to use her bank card or credit cards at the pub.

When she arrived at the bank, there was already another lady using the ATM. So Hazel sorted through her purse, getting her wallet ready while a man looking to be middle-aged came in behind her. She looked up at the man and smiled. He stared ahead without making any eye contact. Hazel thought there was something off about the man but figured it was just her.

The lady ahead of her finished up at the ATM and left. Hazel went up to the machine and put her card into the ATM and started putting in her information. While doing this, she had strong feelings overcome her like something just wasn't quite right. Hazel looked back behind her at the man standing there. He looked away when she looked at him. She turned back to the machine to finish up her transaction when suddenly everything went black.

When Hazel came to, she found herself lying in one of the local parks amongst the trees and bushes, with most of her clothing removed. She became overwhelmed with emotions as she realized that she was a victim of sexual assault. She was left alone in the dark in an area she did not recognize.

When the police arrived, they asked Hazel the usual questions that go along with situations like this. During the questioning, Hazel told the police that she felt something wasn't quite right, but she didn't leave as she didn't want to offend the man plus figured it was just her. She chose to ignore her gut instincts and personal safety to spare the feelings of a stranger.

What are the things that Hazel could have done when she got that gut feeling that something wasn't quite right? I will give you a moment to think about it. Okay, have you come up with an answer or two? Let's see if you and I match up.

When Hazel had these feelings that something was wrong, she could have offered the man to go ahead of her so she could either keep an eye on him or leave the bank as he was using the ATM. Or another option could be to leave right away, saying she forgot something in her car. In both scenarios, she would keep a lookout to make sure the man was not following her.

Don't Think It Can't Happen To You

Most people have this habit of normalcy. They will hear about something awful happening to someone else like a co-worker who lives across town, having their house broken into, and they brush it off as it won't happen to me because that was across town. Bad things can and will happen to anyone without any notice. No matter where or who you are. Falling into the trap of thinking your typical day to day life will remain as is could cost you at some point.

You need to break out of the habit of normalcy and realize that there are potential dangers out there. No need to become paranoid that an attacker is hiding behind every bush, but you need to become aware of potential dangers and how to avoid them. Using these concepts and strategies in this book will help you break the normalcy trap. You will become alert to your surroundings and have improved situational awareness skills. You will develop plans for various scenarios you could encounter.

Survival Mindset

Having a survival mindset is all about doing whatever it takes to survive any given situation where you have to defend your life or the life of someone else. It's about doing what you need to do at the moment without hesitation. Do whatever it takes to get away safely. Push through the fear, pain, and exhaustion that occurs. Allowing just one of those elements to get the better of you, you could lose your life, be assaulted, captured, or someone you care about could die.

Often a victim will succumb to their assailant because they were not mentally tough enough. They allowed the fear of what was happening, or what could happen to them, defeat them mentally. Or they are experiencing a great deal of pain, and they don't know how to overcome or push through it. Mentally they focus on the pain instead of the tasks needed to stop their attacker long enough to escape.

Exhaustion is another factor that will defeat you in a situation where you have to defend off an attacker. Fear, pain, and the dump of adrenaline can tire you out pretty quickly when fighting for your life. Mental toughness and the will to survive is what keeps survivors alive. Some people have this naturally in them, whereas others simply don't. The good news is you can learn it through training. With Martial Arts and self-defense training, you are taught how to deal with each of these elements through drills that build you up.

The main take away from having a survival mindset is to do whatever it takes to stop your assailant long enough for you to escape safely and to get help. Fear, pain, and exhaustion are on the back burner until you and anyone else has escaped safely.

How to Look and Act Confident

Predators hunting for their next potential victim are looking for someone who they perceive as weak and lacking confidence—someone who will be an easy target. Not looking around, not paying attention to their surroundings, keeping their head down, walking, and conducting themselves with a sense of uneasiness or nervousness are just a few of the things that a predator is looking for in their prey. They assume someone like this won't fight back or give them any trouble.

To help reduce the chances of falling victim to a predator, look and act confident. Predators see confident people as harder prey to sneak up on and control. A lot of what a predator is seeking is that control factor. Making their victim do whatever the predator wants without resistance of any kind. So projecting your confidence will help deter a predator from choosing you as their next prey.

But how does one look and act confident? Some people are naturally confident. You look at them, and just by the way they carry themselves and by their body language, you know they have confidence. If you are one of those who needs a little help in this area, don't stress as many people are in the same boat as you. It takes practice.

Some essential tips to help you project confidence even if you aren't

- Be engaged with your surroundings
- Making eye contact with people
- Acknowledging people around you
- Walk tall with shoulders and head up
- Own your personal space around you
- Assertively use your voice when appropriate
- Don't be fidgety
- Speak slowly and clearly
- Allow for silences
- Keep your hands visible
- Take big steps

- Have your personal belongings on you organized

There is also looking and acting too confident to the point where it swings the other way. You appear arrogant, which is another sign of lacking confidence. Predators pick up on this just as easily. So by practicing the tips above and making them subconscious habits, you will appear confident. Over time, your new habits and body language will help build up your confidence. Plus, learning and implementing the concepts and strategies within these pages will empower you to take control of your day to day life, which in return helps build up your confidence as well.

Staying Fit and Strong

Piggybacking off our discussion on looking and acting confident, being physically fit helps you feel confident. When you think of self-defense, it is just not defending yourself from being physically or emotionally harmed by another person. Self-defense is also about defending your health. Within reason obviously. You can't stop the process of aging, but you can slow down the effects by keeping yourself healthy, strong, and fit.

Staying fit and healthy will help you physically fight off and escape from an attack by an assailant. Whether a situation only lasts a few seconds or several minutes, you need to be able to fight the whole time, so your assailant doesn't accomplish whatever they intend to do with you. Being in shape, especially fight shape, allows you to fight through the fear, pain, and exhaustion that you read about earlier.

So besides combating the effects of aging, and allowing you to fight back in a defense situation, looking fit will be another deterrence for predators. Predators are looking for prey that is easy for them to handle. If you look fit and look like you can handle yourself, this will help reduce the risks of being attacked—another tool in your toolbox of self-defense.

RUNNING THE TRAILS

Miesha is a fourth-year university student who loves early morning runs. Especially early mornings on the trails, where the sun shines between the trees, and there's still a bit of a chill in the air. Running early mornings is part of Miesha's daily routine that prepares her for the rest of her day.

It was another beautiful morning on the trails. Early enough that the trails weren't busy yet. Miesha was running at a good pace. Heart pounding in her chest, breathing slightly more focused, and sweat dripping down from her eyebrows. Everyone who would see Miesha on the trails would all agree she looked fit and confident.

Running down the trail, Miesha was taking in the beautiful scenery while smiling and saying hello to everyone she met along the way.

As she approached a more isolated and secluded part of the trail, she noticed there was a man standing alongside the path. The man was wearing a hooded jacket and kept his head down. She didn't feel comfortable with the situation, so she made sure that he knew that she saw him from a distance. She even said good morning to him with a raised voice with confidence as she passed him. Despite that, it was another excellent morning run.

Later that night, Miesha was getting out of shower and towelling herself off when her roommate Sally yelled at her to come here. Miesha went over to the desk where Sally was looking at her laptop. Sally was reading a news article on Facebook about a young college student who had been assaulted earlier in the day on the same running trail where Miesha runs. That's when Miesha realized that she could have been the one assaulted earlier in the morning. Miesha was shocked but also angry at the fact that someone could be so cruel as to assault another human being.

The girls read that the man who assaulted the young lady was already in police custody. The article also mentioned that the police were warning college girls to be more alert by paying attention to their surroundings more, and that predators look for potential victims who are distracted and who look like they lack confidence.

CHAPTER TWO
STRATEGIES TO HELP
AVOID DANGERS

Situational Awareness

Situational awareness is being aware of everything going on around you. You know pretty much everything that is in your immediate area, such as a room you are in, for example. You know who is around you and what those people are doing. What's the mood or atmosphere of the situation you find yourself in, and paying attention to the behaviours and mannerisms of the people you are with. Once you collect all this information, you can make smart decisions on what you should do. In most cases, you won't have too much at all since 99.9% of people are pretty cool and won't harm you. However, by using situational awareness and collecting all the information about everything around you, you can implement the appropriate concepts and strategies in this book. By using the information you have, you can respond to the situation instead of being caught off guard.

Situational awareness is probably one of the most if not the most essential concepts you need to know to avoid dangers of all kinds. Many of the other strategies rely on situational awareness as the first line of defense. So elements of situational awareness will pop up repeatedly within these pages.

Being Aware Of Your Surroundings

When we take out the people in the equation, everything else will be your focus. If we first look at being in a room, for example, you are going to take note of everything.

You will include locations of exits, windows, chairs, tables, items that may become potential weapons for defense, places you can hide, and so on. So if something were to happen, you now have the information you need to make quick decisions on what to do. Can you exit the room safely? Do you need to hide quickly? Will you need to use a chair to strike your assailant so you can get away? All options are available to you because you are aware of your surroundings.

Another example would be you walking down the street, downtown in your city. Lots of people going in and coming out of all the storefronts, traffic is semi-busy on the roads. So lots of distractions going on. You need to be aware of lots of people all around you. Is there anyone who is following you purposely and not just going with the flow of people? What are the people at the traffic lights doing? Where are the questionable alleyways? Where are stores you can go into if you need help? Are there any police officers around, or are you close to a police station? Any potential escape routes you can take?

The Five-Second Rule

The five-second rule is when you enter a new environment, you will take five seconds to look around and take note of everything in your current surroundings. You will look for who is about and what they are doing. Search around for accessible exits in case you need to leave quickly—places to hide if you weren't able to escape or leave the area. Are there any items that could be potential weapons for defense? All the things we discussed in situational awareness and being aware of your surroundings. The five-second rule is the actual habit you constantly use throughout your day.

Now let's use the example of going to the gas station to fill your vehicle. When you are driving up to the gas pump, scan the general area. Is there anyone else filling their vehicle up with gas? Is there anyone just standing around? Do you notice any clear escape routes in case you need to leave the gas station in a hurry to avoid a dangerous situation? Is this a self-serve or full-service station?

As you park your vehicle and shut off the ignition, you take a brief moment to scan the area before you leave your car. What observations are you making? Did anything change from the time you approached the gas station to the time you shut off the ignition? Have you noticed anything new you did not see on your approach?

Exiting your car, you should scan the immediate area around your vehicle as you are filling it with gas. Observe the people around you. Make notes of any exit routes you may need to use. Are there any items nearby that you could you as potential weapons for self-defense? Pay attention to your gut instincts if something feels off. Act on those instincts accordingly and in a timely fashion. You don't want to waste any time if there is a potentially dangerous situation in the making.

If the gas station is self serve and you have to go into the gas bar to pay for gas, take a moment to look in the window of the door before you enter. Does everything look okay? You wouldn't want to walk in on a situation like an argument between the gas attendant and an angry customer. Or perhaps there is a robbery going on that you didn't notice while pumping your gas. It only takes a brief moment to make sure your new environment is safe for you to enter.

At this point, are you done checking everything? Well, actually no. You still need to get back to your vehicle and drive off safely and make sure no one is following you from the gas station. It would be best if you were always using the five-second rule to observe your surroundings without being afraid or paranoid. Use it as one of your tools in your toolbox of self-defense and empowerment.

Situational Awareness Test

The situational awareness test is an excellent way to strengthen your five-second-rule habit. Start the test by entering a new environment that is not as common to you—preferable a crowed meeting room or perhaps a busy lunch court. Take a seat and scan the room for five seconds. Take in as much information as you can. Now close your eyes and try to tell yourself the answers to the following questions.

- What colour is the shirt of the closest person to your left wearing?

- Where is the closest exit to you?

- What is the gender of the person closest to your right?

- What is the item that is closest to you that you could use it as a weapon to defend yourself?

- Where is the closest window in case you had to escape through it?

- Is there somewhere nearby that you could hide behind in an emergency?

Now open your eyes and check to see how many of the questions you answered correctly. The more you practice your situational awareness and the five-second rule with this test, the better you will become. To the point, that becomes second nature for you, and you won't have to put much effort into it, just like breathing or walking.

Don't Wait for Situation to Escalate

Now, this can apply to many different concepts and strategies in this book, but I thought I would cover it now for you, as it will pop up again. Don't wait for the situation to escalate, which most times can happen quite quickly. If you sense that the escalation will become dangerous, you should remove yourself from the situation as soon as you can. Don't wait until it is too late.

Not waiting for the situation to escalate applies to various scenarios. One example would be a large man cornering a woman into the corner of a room yelling and threatening her. If she felt threatened and believed the man was going to strike her or worse, she can pre-emptive hit the man to create space so she can escape the situation without being harmed.

Years ago, a couple of friends were at a house party just down the street from me. While at the party, one of the friends got a weird feeling that something wasn't quite right. They chose to ignore it for a bit but couldn't shake the feeling. So they told their friend that they thought they should go because something wasn't quite right. As they left the house, they were jumped and were dragged off the front porch with their heads banging off the stair steps, and were assaulted in the front yard. Luckily a neighbour happened to be outside and saw the incident occurring and yelled at them to stop. The assailants took off.

It's hard to predict the outcome of any scenario where violence is involved. But when you sense there is something wrong, or you sense the escalation will become violent, remove yourself as quickly as possible. Don't wait for it to be too late.

When I was a young instructor, I knew a young teen girl who had a rough start to life. Her parents weren't the kindest to her, making life pretty rough for her. So she came off rough around the edges and seemed to have issues with authority figures. In spite of the fact she was rude to a lot of her teachers and adults in her life, everyone tried to be patient and help the girl out.

One day the girl got into an altercation with some local teens. I guess she was mouthing off to them and getting right up in their faces over some silly argument. The other teens try to walk away, but she wouldn't let up.

43

Kept right in their faces, enticing them to do something about it. Well, that is precisely what happened. They taught her a hard lesson in not escalating a situation.

Besides not sticking around waiting for a situation to escalate, you don't want to be the cause of the escalation. As you read in the above story, someone might not appreciate what you are doing or trying to do and retaliate.

How The News Can Help You Prepare

The news can help you prepare yourself for self-defense situations. How, you may be thinking. Well, it's no secret that the news, whether it be on television, on the Internet, on the radio, or in the newspapers, loves reporting all the bad things going on. The evening news can be quite depressing if you watch it. Stories of young children who have been shot, a teen girl has gone missing, a college girl has been sexually assaulted on campus, and it goes on. You can use these horrible stories as lessons.

I don't recommend you do this all the time, but every so often, you should pick a few different news stories and learn from them. Go through the following process.

- Select a news story that something horrible has happened to someone—a mugging, for example.

- Does the story describe the events leading up to the mugging? If no, imagine some scenarios that would lead up to the mugging and how you would avoid them. If yes, how would you do things differently?

- Now imagine yourself in the middle of the scenario. What would you do to protect yourself or keep yourself safe?

- Imagine the same scenario, but you are with someone. How does this change up what you would do versus being alone? What are the things you would do differently?

- What are all the things that could go wrong if you were to defend yourself or someone else?

- What emotions are you experiencing when this scenario is "happening" to you?

If you practice this process consistently, you will be mentally preparing yourself for situations you may encounter. You will develop plans for various scenarios that you can respond to instead of reacting to because you were caught off guard. Also, going through the emotions will help you understand how these emotions will affect what you do when you are in the moment. This process will help you be more in control when and if something happens.

Have a Plan

As you just read, the news is a powerful tool for preparing yourself for various situations where you may have to defend yourself. After you have gone through the exercise where you go through different scenarios and what you would do and how you would feel, you now have to have plans for these situations. It is a simple process to develop these plans.

First, write down a list of all the situations that could happen to you. Each person will have a different list based on various factors. Such factors may include; where they live, married with kids or not, living in a house versus an apartment, commuting to work in a car versus taking public transit, and so on.

An example list could include:

- Being mugged at the ATM

- Being followed by a stranger on the bus

- Being assaulted while alone in the elevator. with a stranger

- Being grabbed while jogging in the local park

- A friend has had something slipped into their drink at a party

- Someone corners you in the dorm

- You are at the movie theatre, and an active shooter comes in firing away

- Being held at gunpoint when you have your kids with you

- Someone is trying to carjack you while your kids are in the backseat of the car

Now once you have compiled your list, it's time to go through each scenario and write out a plan on what you will do if this happens. Now write out for each situation what you can do to help reduce the risks of this happening to you. Some situations may be entirely out of your control. People are people; you cannot control what they will do. Lastly, for each scenario, write out what you are going to do after the fact. What do you need to do and who do you need to contact.

Once you have all this written out, you now need to engrave these plans into your subconscious. So if something happens, you can respond with your plan. Also, share your plans with other people you are regularly with, so they know what to do if a situation were to occur while with you. Situations will happen so fast that you won't have time to communicate with anyone amid the chaos effectively. Best to be prepared ahead of time with good solid plans. One more quick note on this. Your plans probably won't play out exactly like you envisioned. You will have to adapt on the spot.

Avoid Potentially Dangerous Situations

One of the best defenses is don't be there. If you are not there, there won't be any need to physically defending yourself. That is pretty close to what avoiding potentially dangerous situations is. You need to dig in a bit further, though. It's just not about avoiding something or someplace physically. It is about seeing what could go wrong and act in a way that will help reduce the risks of something happening.

Here is a sample list of potentially dangerous situations and what you can do to avoid them:

- Being carjacked while sitting at red light

  - Make sure your car doors are locked, and windows are up while driving

- Being pulled into the bushes and sexually assaulted while you were running late at night on the running trails

  - Run during the daytime or run in a well lit and very public visible area

- Someone slipped something into your drink at a party, and you end up in a bedroom alone with someone you don't know

  - Keep your hands and eyes on your drink at all times, and get your own drinks instead of someone else

- You got punched in the face while in a heated argument

  - Stay calm in all situations, so things don't escalate, and if they are escalating, remove yourself from the situation until things calm down

Now add to this list. What are the potentially dangerous situations that you could find yourself in, and how can you help avoid them? As you are discovering, preventing potentially dangerous situations from occurring in the first place is one of our main goals in self-defense. Rationally you are defending yourself all the time.

Years ago, a bunch of my friends and I went to another's friend's house for a dinner party. It was a good night of friends and lots of tasty foods. One of our friends brought one of her other guy friends from outside our regular circle of friends. He broke up with his girlfriend, and she thought he would like to get out of the house and meet some new people. He seemed like an okay guy.

As the evening progressed, he became very aggressive with the ladies. At first, just playfully hitting on them. But when no one was falling for his charms, he got irate and started threatening everyone. At this point, he was heavily intoxicated. The night progressed, as you can imagine.

When it was time to leave, my friend was taking a few of us plus her other friend, who was being quite the challenge home after the party. He was very out of control and aggressive in the car as well. To the point that one of our other friends and he got into a bit of a verbal confrontation to put it politely. Needless to say, I was not impressed and was ready to kick him out of the vehicle. My friend planned to drop everyone off before taking this guy home.

I told her she should drop him off first even if it meant taking more time to drop the rest of us off afterwards. I didn't feel comfortable leaving her in the car with this angry guy. I know for a fact she can handle herself, but why risk it if you don't have to. I'd rather avoid a potentially harmful situation before it even gets the chance to start. She agreed and dropped him off at his apartment before taking the rest of us home.

Escape Routes

Escape routes will come up in later sections of this book in the appropriate concepts and strategies; however, I wanted to mention it here briefly as well. Escape routes allow you to escape a situation after you have had to defend yourself from an assailant, or it can be your avenue of escape from a potential situation.

In the case where you had to defend yourself from an attack while caught off guard, this is where you would escape to safety. It could mean you run into a nearby business for help. You escape and lock yourself in a room where your attacker cannot get in while you call for help. You put a physical barrier between you and your attacker until you can escape or help comes, and many more. Being aware of your surroundings enables you to find these escape routes faster than you would without practicing situational awareness or making use of the five-second rule.

Another scenario could be that you are walking down the street and notice that a stranger is following you. Your intuition is letting you know something may be off. Again you could go into a local business nearby and see if the stranger continues to walk past or do they come in the store looking for you. In that case, you may want to ask for help. You could cross the street and see if they do the same. Crossing the street and walking in the direction you came from to observe their reaction. In all cases, having your phone ready in case you need to call for help. Also, there are many other options available to you. All depends on where you are.

A NIGHT OUT WITH THE GIRLS

It started like any other typical Friday night for university kids. Always a party or social gathering to attend. This Friday night was no different. Miesha, Sally, and a few of their girlfriends were going to a local pub for drinks and a good time. Miesha and Sally were meeting their friends at the pub after Miesha got off work from the law firm where she worked as an intern.

Miesha and Sally met up with their friends shortly after 9 pm. It was apparent when the two girls arrived that the other girls had already started to have a good time without them. A few of them already seemed to be a tad tipsy from the shots of vodka consumed before Miesha and Sally arrived. Both girls were not much into the drinking scene except for the occasional beer when they went out for a bite to eat with a group of friends.

One of their friends, Nora, on the other hand, is the exact opposite. She enjoys the vodka shots a little more than the average person does to put it politely. This night was no different. While the girls were sitting around their table enjoying the drinks and munching on some appetizers, a group of college boys entered the pub. At first sight, you could tell a few of the boys amongst the group were cocky and full of themselves. Thinking they were god's gift to the world with their loud look at me mannerism.

It wasn't long before the two groups starting mingling. One of the young men in the group caught Miesha's attention as he was sitting back from the group and observing everything that was going on, not saying much. Intrigued, she walked over and introduced herself to him, as she was similar in settings like this. "My name is Miesha," she said. "Hey, My name is Logan," he responded. "Would you care to join me?" She accepted his offer.

They sat back and watched the girls and boys from their groups mingle and having a good time. No drinks were left unturned. Everyone seemed to be enjoying each other's company. Nora went over to the bar to grab herself another couple of shots, where she met Tyson, one of the boys from Logan's group of friends. They started talking, and soon enough, Tyson asked Nora if she wanted to go outside to get some air, which she said she would love to.

Nora, who was overly intoxicated and Tyson, left the pub together. Observing them, both Miesha and Logan got a gut feeling that something wasn't quite right. So Miesha, lead by Logan, went outside to see if they could see where Nora and Tyson had gone. Miesha and Logan could not see them, so they started to head down the street in hopes they would find them.

Suddenly there was a loud cry coming from the alley ahead. Logan took off running towards the direction of the bellow with Miesha firmly behind him. As they entered the alleyway, Logan saw Tyson restraining Nora against the wall. She was struggling to get away and pleading with Tyson to stop. Logan rushed over and grabbed Tyson by the shoulders and pulled him away from Nora. Tyson turned around, facing Logan and swung at him. Logan blocked Tyson's wild punch and delivered one of his own to Tyson's solar plexus causing him to collapse to the ground gasping for air.

Miesha rushed over and pulled Nora away from the scene. Nora was distraught, telling Miesha that she told

Tyson to stop, but he wouldn't listen. He forced himself on to Nora and disregarded her wishes. Shortly after, the police arrived and arrested Tyson for attempted sexual assault.

CHAPTER THREE
WHEN YOU HAVE TO DEFEND YOURSELF

O kay, now let's talk about when you actually have to defend yourself physically from an assault. Assuming you did everything correctly when trying to avoid all potentially dangerous situations, an attack can still happen. It happens all the time. In fact, every 90 seconds, one violent crime was committed in Canada according to the statistics for 2018. That number in the United States of America was 2.3 violent crimes every 60 seconds.

With those kinds of numbers, it is imperative you learn the following concepts and strategies in this section. They will equip you with some tools to help ensure your safety and escape from your assailant. One key thing you must understand is that you must be willing to do anything necessary to stop the attack and escape the situation immediately.

The following is an excerpt from the Government of Canada Justice Laws Website: https://laws.justice.gc.ca/eng/acts/C-46/page-7.html#h-115831

Defence of Person

Defence — use or threat of force

34 (1) A person is not guilty of an offence if

(a) they believe on reasonable grounds that force is being used against them or another person or that a threat of force is being made against them or another person;

(b) the act that constitutes the offence is committed for the purpose of defending or protecting themselves or the other person from that use or threat of force; and

(c) the act committed is reasonable in the circumstances.

Factors

(2) In determining whether the act committed is reasonable in the circumstances, the court shall consider the relevant circumstances of the person, the other parties and the act, including, but not limited to, the following factors:

(a) the nature of the force or threat;

(b) the extent to which the use of force was imminent and whether there were other means available to respond to the potential use of force;

(c) the person's role in the incident;

(d) whether any party to the incident used or threatened to use a weapon;

(e) the size, age, gender and physical capabilities of the parties to the incident;

(f) the nature, duration and history of any relationship between the parties to the incident, including any prior use or threat of force and the nature of that force or threat;

(f.1) any history of interaction or communication between the parties to the incident;

(g) the nature and proportionality of the person's response to the use or threat of force; and

(h) whether the act committed was in response to a use or threat of force that the person knew was lawful.

No defence

(3) Subsection (1) does not apply if the force is used or threatened by another person for the purpose of doing something that they are required or authorized by law to do in the administration or enforcement of the law, unless the person who commits the act that constitutes the offence believes on reasonable grounds that the other person is acting unlawfully.

- R.S., 1985, c. C-46, s. 34
- 1992, c. 1, s. 60(F)
- 2012, c. 9, s. 2

If you live in another country, please check with your local laws pertaining to your laws on self-defense.

Use Your Voice

Don't be afraid to use your voice to draw attention to the situation and/or command the attacker to stop what they are doing. The louder you are, the better. Firstly, this may deter the assailant from continuing with their assault because they don't want others to see what is going on. Rarely does a predator wish to be seen, so they pick victims they think will not draw attention to them.

Secondly, using your voice in a loud and confident fashion may repel the attacker from continuing with their assault on you. You are showing them your strength and willingness to fight back. Again most predators pick their victims because they see them as easy prey. Most of them won't want to fight. However, there is always the exception to the rule. You may end up with an assailant who doesn't care about how much of a fight you put up.

Don't Be Afraid To Cause A Scene

Similar to using your voice to deter an attacker, you can't be afraid to cause a scene. Again most predators usually go after victims they think will be easy for them to control. Being loud and animated, causing as much commotion as possible to attract attention to you and your attacker may cause the attacker to flee the scene or change what they are doing.

If your attacker flees the scene, you need to do the same and get help and tell them what just happened. If your attacker doesn't take off but is startled by your reaction, you now have an advantage. While they are momentarily startled, you can use your strikes to stop their attacks and escape the situation.

Remove Yourself From The Situation As Fast As Possible

Never, and I mean never, stay around after you have successfully defended off your assailant. You need to leave as fast as possible. If your attacker flees the scene because they don't want to get caught or you successfully fought them off, you need to leave as well in case they come back for you.

If you find yourself in a situation where you have successfully incapacitated your assailant, you need to leave the scene. Don't stick around to admire your handy work. Your assailant may recover quickly and come after you. So once you have done what is needed to stop the attack, you leave right away and go get help and tell them what just happened. Always report any incident where you had to defend yourself, whether it was physical or not.

Protect Your Head

When you find yourself in the midst of being struck by your attacker, cover up your head. Your head is the most important thing you need to protect. There are a lot of sensitive areas that can easily be severely damaged by wild punches. It only takes one well-placed strike to the head to cause death. Less severe blows can still blind you, cause you to lose hearing, create breathing issues, cause you to lose consciousness, and so on.

You need to cover up your head with your hands and arms. One of the best ways to cover up your head is to grab the back of your skull at the base with your hands. Now try to squeeze your elbows together, causing your arms to cover up your ears, temples, eyes, nose, and jaw. Now tuck your chin down and into your chest to help protect the chin, neck, and throat.

Your arms are extremely tough, especially the elbows. Most people will end up hurting their hands on your arms if they continue to strike at your head. If any punches happen to land on your elbows, most likely the attacker will break the small bones in their hand, quite a common injury actually.

Protecting your head this way will help reduce the risk of injuries while keeping you conscious and alert. Covering up your head will provide you with time to figure out what you need to do to stop your assailant from assaulting you.

Know Their Weaknesses

Earlier in the book, we covered your strengths. Now it is time to go over your potential attacker's weaknesses and use your strengths against them. Some easy vital targets on the body are: eyes, ears, nose, throat, groin, solar plexus, kidneys, and knees.

The eyes are super sensitive. Striking or poking them with the fingers and thumbs can cause a lot of pain and blindness. Striking the ears with palm strikes, hammer fists, slaps, punches, or elbows will cause pain and a loss of balance and orientation. Hitting the nose with virtually any strike can break it, causing pain and difficulty in breathing. The throat is very sensitive, as well. Striking this area can create extreme difficulty in breathing and even death.

Striking the solar plexus with a hard punch, kick, knee, or elbow can cause a great deal of pain and make it hard to breathe. Hitting the kidneys has similar effects to striking the solar plexus. Kicking the front, side, or back of the knees can severely damage them and cause your attacker not to be able to stand up or walk. Now the one you have been waiting for, the groin. A well-placed strike to the groin, especially a good kick or knee, is simply crippling. I know this first hand.

I have been kicked in the groin on many occasions while sparring and conducting self-defense workshops for women. The hardest blow I ever received to the groin was in early September on a Thursday morning about five years ago as of this writing of this book. I literally curled up into the fetal position and had tears in my eyes. I was utterly helpless. There would have been no way I could have defended myself at that moment.

You will find when practicing the various combative strikes used for self-defense that you will naturally lean towards certain techniques. Pay attention to this. The techniques that you seem to do more often will be the ones you do in a real-life situation. Use this knowledge to develop your striking strategies and strengths.

Don't Be Relocated

Sometimes an attacker will try to relocate their victim for whatever purpose they may have for them. Under no circumstances do you allow the assailant to relocate or take you away. The chances of surviving an encounter with an assailant who takes you away drops down next to zero chances. You are safer where you are when the encounter starts.

You need to do whatever it takes to avoid being relocated by your attacker. Use all the tactics in this book to ensure your safety and survival.

What Is The Real Danger

So being attacked, grabbed, followed, threatened, and so forth are all dangerous. There are different degrees of danger. Some are low risk, while others are much higher risk. But what I want to discuss is what is the real danger in any given encounter. It might be different than what you think. You need to establish immediately what are the real threats that you have to deal with first.

The best way to explain this is with a few examples. First example, if someone grabs your wrist in a threatening matter while in a heated argument. What is the real danger or threat? Most people would say the hand that is grabbing your wrist. Well, not really. Yes, it is unpleasant; however, grabbing your wrist won't really do much to you. It may hurt a bit, but that's about it. I would be more concerned if the attacker were trying to pull you somewhere or if the other hand was going to strike you. In this case, you should try to break their wrist grab so you can escape, or neutralize the other arm, so they can't hit you with it. Being grabbed is far safer than being hit.

The second example is your assailant is choking you with two hands. What is the real danger or threat in this situation for you? The risk is losing consciousness due to a lack of oxygen from your assailant's hands choking your neck. Being choked is far more dangerous compared to the first example of being grabbed on the wrist. You need to free your neck and throat from your attacker's hands immediately. This is a top priority, then disable your attacker so you can get away quickly and safely.

In any encounter where you may have to defend yourself, you need to recognize what the real immediate dangers are so you can deal with them first. Dealing with the wrong things first can have severe consequences for you.

Self-Defense Weapons and Tools

Now, this is a tricky topic. Here in Canada, you are technically not allowed to carry anything with the intent to use it as a weapon for self-defense. I would check with the local laws in your country. Some countries allow you to carry various items such as pepper spray, mace, and even a firearm, amongst other items.

You could carry a kubaton keychain. It is a keychain generally made out of light aluminium. It allows you to strike with the keys in a cutting action as you swing it at your attacker's face. You can also use it to poke your attacker with the blunt end making your hammer fist strikes way more effective compared to normal.

Another option is to carry a tactical pen. A tactical pen is just a pen that you can write with that is reinforced on the inside to make it stronger, allowing for a strong stabbing and poking weapon. Simply by looking at a tactical pen versus a regular pen, you won't be able to notice the difference.

What Can You Use As A Potential Weapon

The reality is the attacker may be too big and strong for you to handle, and you may need to resort to using a weapon to defend yourself. If you don't carry a self-defense weapon or tool on your person, you will need to find something in the immediate area to use as a weapon. But what can you use? The answer is anything you can get a hold of that will cause pain or damage to your attacker. As long as you can handle it and use it effectively against your attacker, use it.

Note on using any sort of weapon against an attacker: You run the risk of having your assailant take the weapon away from you and use it on you. So be prepared for that scenario. Another thing I want to mention is it takes a lot of training to use weapons effectively. If you think you will need to use a weapon, make sure you get proper training for it.

SELF DEFENSE SEMINAR

Graduation is less then a month away. The students are busy with final assignments; studying for upcoming exams, and the last few events they will all take part in together. Miesha and Sally have been roommates for their entire university career. They are looking forward to their new lives outside of school.

Miesha was looking through the weekly university newspaper when she came across a notice for a self-defense seminar for the female students this upcoming Friday night at the school gymnasium. She asked Sally if she would like to attend with her. Sally replied, "Yeah, it sounds like fun. With all the things that have happened this year, it's probably a good idea to learn some moves."

Miesha and Sally arrived at the school gymnasium early to warm up a bit and stretch out before the self-defense workshop started. Before the workshop got started, Miesha mentioned to Sally how there weren't that many ladies there. She thought there would have been more attendees as she believed all women should learn how to protect themselves.

The instructors of the workshop started by going over various tips and concepts for the first ten minutes, strategies that would help keep women safe by avoiding dangerous situations before they occur in the first place. They emphasized that ninety percent of self-defense is mental and ten percent physical. The last ten percent was for last resort only. They stressed that the seminar attendees should focus on their mental strategies just as much as their physical techniques they would be learning tonight.

Now for the good stuff, the secret death touch, one-finger takedowns, ripping the balls off, and getting out the ninja stars, thought Sally. Well, not exactly. No secrets or fancy moves were taught. The instructors taught Miesha and the other girls how powerful they were using some basic strikes. Such strikes as elbows, knees, palms, and basic kicks with the feet and shins.

Miesha and Sally noticed that a lot of the defense techniques the instructors were teaching were relatively the same basic techniques from various situations. Techniques as elbow strikes, palm strikes, knee strikes, stomps, and low kicks. These basic techniques will help to defend yourself from bear hugs, chokes, wrist grabs, hair grabs, and so on. Going back to their dorm room after the workshop, both Sally and Miesha felt confident that they had the tools and knowledge to defend themselves if the need ever came up.

CHAPTER FOUR
LEARNING SELF DEFENSE

Now you have some excellent ideas on what your strengths are, what your attacker's weaknesses are, and what weapons you can use. You also are drilling in the habits of practicing situational awareness and having plans already worked out in case an assailant ever attacks you. You may be wondering what is next?

Getting some hands-on training is the next step. You could do everything right when it comes to avoiding dangerous situations, and you could still find yourself confronted with an assailant. You read up on the previous section on how to use your strengths against your assailant's weaknesses. You know a bit about using self-defense weapons. You know to leave the scene of the attack as soon as you can and to report the incident afterward. Now you need to get your hands dirty.

Take A Self Defense Course

A good starting point after you have read some good books on self-defense, such as this one, is to take a self-defense course or workshop. Courses can vary in length from a one-week course to 6 weeks or more where they teach you basic combative strikes and how to defend against various attacks. These are good to take. You will also find 2-hour self-defense workshops where they teach you the basics. Generally, these courses are a good preview on how that instructor(s) or martial arts academy teaches their self-defense.

You want to find a course or workshop that covers the scenarios you are most concerned with. Meaning you would probably not sign up for a class where they teach you how to become an escape artist from handcuffs. Unless that is your thing or you are auditioning to become the next Bond girl. Also, you wouldn't be signing up for a course where they teach you about military tactics in the jungle if you are a mother of three living in a small town and not travelling to the jungle.

You want to find the course that covers the topics you want to learn about. The easiest way is to contact the instructor or martial arts academy that is conducting the courses or workshops and ask them questions about what they will be teaching. Let them know what your concerns and interests are. If it's a good fit for you, they will let you know. Any reputable academy will let you know if what they teach is not right for your needs.

Take Up Martial Arts

Now I may be a little biased on this one, but I strongly recommend taking up martial arts. Besides the obvious self-defense benefits you will be gaining and practicing, martial arts provides a wealth of other benefits. Such benefits include improving your strength and power, increased cardiovascular conditioning and endurance, flexibility and mobility training, confidence building, a way to manage stress, making new friends, and much more.

But what martial arts style should you learn? Well, that will depend on your goals. If you are taking up martial arts for strictly self-defense, look for academies that emphasize self-defense. If you are seeking more for a sports martial arts school, then find one you like. There are also a lot of schools that do both. These are your best options. They give you more variety in what you will learn, and your training will be more enjoyable.

When searching for a martial arts academy, you must know whether you want a stand-up/striking style, a ground/grappling style, or a school that teaches both. Stand up/striking styles teach their students how to use their hands, arms, elbows, feet, shins, and knees to fight and defend themselves. Ground/grappling styles teach their students how to do joint locks, manipulations, and chokes on the ground. These are very brief descriptions as I can write entire chapters on each style, but I want you to get a bit of an idea of what they are.

Then some martial arts academies teach a mixture of both. You may find this appealing as most people do. You get a well-rounded martial arts education that covers all areas of the arts instead of just one specific area. This is important, as you never know what you will need to do in a real-life scenario against an assailant. Our Taekwondo academy teaches a mixture of modern and traditional Taekwondo mixed with a blend of Kickboxing, Jiu-Jitsu, Kabudo, Kali, and Krav Maga. This helps to prepare our students for a wide variety of scenarios that could happen.

Issues With Martial Arts

If you do your research, you will come across books, articles, and videos of "experts" that claim that martial arts training doesn't teach you how to defend yourself. On the one hand, I will say they are correct, and on the other hand, they don't know what they are talking about.

Let me start by defending the "experts" who say that martial arts won't teach you to protect yourself. Most of the time, they are referring to the styles that only practice for sport. Whether that is for in-ring competition via striking like boxing, kickboxing, or sparring or via submission grappling or wrestling. Their primary focus for training is to train only the techniques they can use in competition under controlled rules to ensure the safety of the competitors.

They also refer to the martial arts competitors that compete in forms, weapons, or breaking competitions. These competitions are based on competitors performing their routines or breaks solo. They are not physically competing against or making contact with someone else. They are scored based on how "perfectly" they can perform the techniques. In breaking, you win by who can break the most pine boards or concrete blocks with a single strike.

Rarely does a martial artist only practice one element of their style and never apply it to any self-defense training. This would make them not competent in defending themselves. But this is very rare as most martial artists who train for competition also train for self-defense. Martial Arts, in its purest form, are for combat and self-defense.

However, I will say that some styles will get a bad reputation of being not effective in real-life situations. This happens when practitioners of a school become stuck in the mindset of following the rules of their style. Instead, their focus should be on how they can use the physical tools and strategies of their style to defend against assailants who don't follow the rules.

Martial Arts training will teach you how to defend yourself against various grabs, chokes, strikes, kicks, takedowns, and weapons. Most importantly you will learn how to reduce the risks of being attacked or getting into a confrontation with someone else. This is accomplished through training techniques and drills that help you to develop situational awareness, recognize body language and movements, improve your reaction and respond time, control your emotional responses, and have the best plans for you against various encounters with assailants. Plus Martial Arts is a great way to get in and stay in shape.

Fitness Kickboxing

Fitness Kickboxing is an excellent workout that incorporates a lot of the basic strikes from the Martial Arts as well as a variety of strength and cardiovascular training. If you are looking for a workout that is fun and burns a lot of calories, I cannot recommend fitness kickboxing enough. It's a great workout where you can practice the strikes that you would use to defend yourself.

If you weren't necessarily interested in starting a Martial Arts program right away, you could join an academy that offers both Fitness Kickboxing and self-defense. You can join their fitness kickboxing classes and take part in their self-defense workshops when they are offered. This will allow you to enjoy the fitness side of Martial Arts as well as practice your defense skills to keep them fresh in your mind. Gradually work yourself into joining Martial Arts. You won't regard it.

Self Defense Versus Fighting

Quick note here, you need to understand the difference between self-defense versus fighting. Self-defense occurs when you defend yourself against an attack from an assailant who expects you not to fight back. They would not have attacked you if they thought you might retaliate against their actions ot intents.

Fighting is when two people are challenging each other to see who has superior combat skills. A lot of times, a situation that started out as self-defense can turn into a full out fight. This is what you want to avoid at all costs because you could get seriously hurt, injured, or worst.

There are a few ways that a defense scenario can turn into a fight. One, the person who is being attacked makes it a battle by challenging skills versus skills instead of defending and removing themselves from the situation as quickly as possible. Two, the person who's on defense puts their fists up like a boxer or challenges the assailant to fight, causing their brain to switch over to fight mode. Precisely what you do not want.

What you want is for your assailant to assume you are vulnerable and won't put up a fight. Once they have dropped their guard a bit, you will strike fast and hard, attacking their weaknesses that we discussed earlier. Once the opportunity arises for you to make your escape, you do so as quickly as possible. Once in the clear, report the incident to the authorities.

Act Out Self Defense Scenarios

Like anything else you want to get good at in life, self-defense skills take time and lots of practice to develop to the point that your skills become proficient. So when you are not taking your Martial Arts classes or self-defense workshops, you should act out self-defense scenarios. Find a partner to train with and go over various attacks you could encounter and practice defending yourself from these attacks. Using different locations in and around your home and elsewhere can add variety to your training. The more variety you put into your practicing, the more prepared you will become for unpredictable situations.

IT'S TIME TO LEAVE

Miesha was rushing around the house, getting ready to go out. She was super excited as she was meeting Sally for dinner and it felt like forever since they had seen each other. It had been a few years since they graduated from university, got jobs, and moved in with their boyfriends. Life was busy as responsible adults.

After graduating, Miesha got hired at a local advertising agency. She enjoyed the various projects that she got to work on and made a few new friends. Life was going well. Sally got a job with the municipality office working as a clerk. She spent her days dealing with people, in between her managers giving her tasks to do, and dealing with complaints from the community. Like Miesha, Sally had moved in with her boyfriend, and they got engaged a few months prior.

Miesha and Sally were meeting at a restaurant downtown that used to be their favourite spot to eat and relax when they were in university together. Miesha arrived first and had a hostess seat her at the same table where she and Sally would sit during their university days. She ordered herself a drink while waiting for Sally to arrive. Sipping on her drink, Miesha waved at Sally as she entered the restaurant looking around for Miesha.

Miesha and Sally exchanged pleasantries as they looked over the menus, which had a lot of changes made to them since the ladies were there last. Just like the last time they saw each other, a lot had changed. Miesha told Sally all about her job at the advertising firm, described how cute her new house is, and a bit about her boyfriend. When it was Sally's turn, she kept it brief. Miesha sense something was off with Sally. She seemed different, somehow.

"Okay, you seem not quite yourself. What's up?" Miesha asked. "Everything is fine," "I don't believe you. We were roommates for four years. I know when something is up!" "Just life in general," Sally replied. "Work is stressful." "Work can be stressful from time to time for all of us. You sure there's not something else that is bothering you?" Miesha probed Sally further. "Well...

maybe I shouldn't say anything?!" "Sally, you can tell me anything. You know that, right?" "Yeah, I know. Well, you have to promise me not to say anything to anyone else," Sally replied.

"No matter what I seem to do lately, I can't seem to please my fiancée. He will come home from work upset, and I try to make him feel better, but we end up arguing. I try to relate to him, but he puts down my work. He gets mad at me when I don't have dinner ready for him, or if I don't have the laundry done." Sally went on. "It's worse when he has been drinking. He will call me a bitch or something. It makes me feel like I am worthless." "That's not good, Sally. Why are you putting up with this?" Miesha asked. "Because I know he loves me and I love him." "But people who love each other don't act like that. He is abusive to you." "He's not abusive," Sally replied. "Sounds like it to me. It just doesn't have to be physical for it to be abuse. Has he ever got physical with you?" Miesha asked. "No, no... He has never hit me before."

The rest of the conversation was quiet over dinner. Miesha and Sally finished up dinner, paid their bills and said goodbye to each other. Miesha went home feeling sad for her friend. Sally went home worried that someone was going to find out what she had told Miesha over dinner. If her boyfriend ever found out what she said to Miesha, he would not be pleased. What Sally didn't tell Miesha was that her boyfriend had been physical with her. He hadn't hit Sally but had restrained her against the wall, or held her down on the bed, and a few other incidents.

"Where were you?" Sally's boyfriend said as she came through the front door. "I went out for dinner with Miesha. I told you yesterday I was." "You weren't here to fix my dinner. I have been sitting here waiting for you to come home to cook my dinner." "I'm sorry. I will get at it once I change my clothes." "You will do it right now, woman," he snapped at Sally. "And you better not have told your chick friend about anything... did you?" Sally looked down at her feet, feeling ashamed. "You bitch!" he yelled as he slapped her across the face.

CHAPTER FIVE
RELATIONSHIPS, DATING, AND BEING SOCIAL

Not all violent encounters will happen with random strangers who want your money, out on the running trails, or late nights alone in the parking lot at work. 80% of assailants are friends or are relatives of their victims. Over 50% of offenders are married or in long-term relationships. 80% of sexual assaults happen at home. Over 50% of women in Canada have experienced physical or sexual violence at last once. Once a week, a woman is killed by her intimate partner.

Scary statistics, right? Well, as you just read, the chance of you being assaulted by someone you may know is pretty high. Almost making relationships, dating, and being social a little unsettling. But like mentioned before,

99% of people are pretty cool and you don't have to worry about them. The concepts and strategies in this section will help you avoid and prepare for the other 1%.

Checking In When Going Out With Someone New

In today's world, a lot of people are meeting each other online with online dating sites and dating apps on their smart phones. Anyone can be anyone online as there is no face-to-face contact. So it is hard to really know someone until you decide to go out on that first date.

Essentially you are going out with a complete stranger who you never met before. You have no idea what they are like or what their intentions are. Again, 99% of people are cool, but what if you run into that 1% who wanted to do something unspeakable to you? Would anyone know what happened to you?

You should have a friend who you must check in with while out on the date, as well as when you get home safely. You can be the person who initiates the check-ins by texting or calling your friend. Or your friend can check in on you. If you don't reply within a predetermined time, your friend has your permission to call you or take any further actions you both agreed upon before the date.

This tip is also an excellent tip to use when you have met someone new in person until you get to know that person a bit better. Better to be safe than sorry. Plus, it gives you and your friend something to talk about.

Since I run a Martial Arts academy and have had plenty of female students and ladies attending our empowerment workshops, I hear about a lot of what's going on in the dating scene. More than I probably want to know about sometimes. Anyway, more than a few times, I have had female clients who wanted me to act as a bodyguard for them. By being nearby while they go out on a date with some guy who they weren't sure about, and wanted me to let them know if I thought the guy was safe.

My first response to the first client was, "Sure for $500," To which they responded with "okay." So then I kindly explained to them that if they felt that something was wrong with the guy to the point that they needed a bodyguard around, it was probably not a good idea in the first place. They agreed with me.

Have Someone Watching Out For You

Having someone watching out for you isn't a bad idea, though. You don't need to pay $500 either. When you and your friends go out to parties, pubs, and any social gathering, it's a good idea to watch out for each other. Making sure no one messes with your drinks. Going to the washroom together, making sure no one goes outside alone with a stranger, checking out that person you met, and so on. Little things to help keep each other stay safe.

Years ago a bunch of us adult black belts and older teen black belts were invited to a surprise birthday party. At this party there was a guy who I have never met before. He was highly intoxicated. He was trying to act all cool and being overly vocal and telling these outrageously untrue stories trying to impress all the girls. Two of these girls were two of my students who I have known these since forever and would do anything to protect them.

I didn't like how he was acting towards them—a little too close for comfort. A short while later, a bunch of the younger ones went into the basement of the house to hang out. Of course, me being the father-like figure didn't trust the fact this guy was in the basement with these girls. They weren't alone as others were down there too but I still felt uneasy about it.

I wasn't too worried about the girls if they stuck together. They are black belts, so they know how to handle themselves. In fact I would have loved to see them mop the floors with him. But anyway, you can never be too careful. Unknown to me at the time, a few of my younger male students were there, keeping an eye on things. They told me the next day that they didn't trust this guy either.

When I was leaving the party with a few other people, I texted the girls, letting them know I was going and to let me know when they left, so I knew they were safe. They texted me back, saying they were leaving as well because they didn't feel comfortable being left there alone.

It was nice to see that the girls had other black belts keeping an eye out for them in case something happened. Again these girls can handle themselves, but we would all be a little safer if we would watch out for each other.

Going Outside Alone With Someone You Just Met

Now it is quite natural for you to want to be alone with someone you have just met, and there's this connection. You want to go somewhere where it is quiet, and you can be alone without all the distractions of everything else going on. It's a fantastic feeling. However, is it the safest thing you can do? It all depends on the situation.

You have to look at different factors and decide for yourself if you feel it is safe for you to go outside alone with this person you just met. Are you in the right state of mind to make decisions? If you have been drinking, are you intoxicated? Can you let someone like a friend know that you are going outside to be alone with this person? Do you have your phone with you? If something goes wrong, are you capable of defending yourself or yell for help? Will there be other people outside? There's a good chance everything will be fine, but be prepared to take action if needed.

Recognize Controlling Behaviours

I decided to put this here in this section. Still, the same principles apply when dealing with anyone, including strangers you have never met before.

I knew a lady who was divorcing her husband because of how abusive he was. Not physically but verbally. He would put her down, not in front of anyone but behind closed doors. He was also very controlling. He had to win every argument, and you weren't allowed to bring up past mistakes he made. It was perfectly okay for him to bring up your past mistakes, though, even if it had nothing to do with the current situation.

He was also very controlling and abusive towards their young children. Not allowing them to do anything they wanted or just to let them be children. Being controlled twenty-four hours a day, seven days a week got old after a while, and she demanded a divorce. This was no way to live her life nor for her children. Of course, he didn't understand why. Why shouldn't she want to live this way?

When they were legally divorced, she wanted him to move out until the house was sold. He wouldn't do that even when she offered to buy the other half of the house from him. Nope, he forced her to sell the house. When the house was sold, and they were living in two separate places, he still wanted to know everything she did. He was not getting the picture.

Eventually, all this stopped when she met another guy who eventually would go on to be her husband. Her new marriage is the exact opposite of her previous marriage.

The ability to recognize controlling behaviours can help you avoid troubles before they happen. Controlling behaviours can lead to abusive traits in certain people—

something you want to avoid in relationships and with people in general. Some tells of controlling behaviours include:

- Giving or seeking more attention than normally

- Putting you down when things don't go their way

- Making you feel unworthy or worthless

- Isolating you from friends and family

- Chronic criticism towards you

- Threatening you

- Using guilt as a tool

- Creating a debt, you owe them

- Requiring constant disclosure

- Providing too many details

- Not respecting your time alone

- Not respecting your personal space

- Pressuring you to do something you don't want to do

Use these traits to recognize controlling behaviours in potentially dangerous strangers you encounter as well as any relationships you have or are in. Early detection will help keep you safe from situations you don't want to find yourself in.

It was a beautiful sunny afternoon in the city—lots of people out and about. Nikki, a recent young graduate of the local university, had just picked up some groceries and was heading home. Carrying two big bags full of groceries as she walked through the central park to enjoy some of the scenery. She sat down on one of the park benches to give her arms some rest from carrying the heavy groceries.

After a few moments of enjoying the views of the park, she continued on her way back to her apartment. Dodging in and out of the crowds all over the streets and sidewalks. The city seemed to be much busier with newcomers lately. The front door to Nikki's apartment building required an access code to unlock it. So Nikki placed her groceries on the ground in front of her to punch in the code. The buzzer went off, indicating the door was unlocked. Nikki bent over to pick up her groceries when a voice behind her asked if she needed any help. Slightly startled by the voice, she turned to look up at the man standing there.

"No, that's okay. Thanks for the offer," replied Nikki as she picked up her groceries off the ground. "They aren't too heavy." "But I insist." said the man as he reached for one of Nikki's bags. "Which floor do you live on?" Nikki pulled the bag back a bit and again thanked the man for his offer. She opened the door and headed towards the evaluator. The man followed Nikki, making small talk. Telling her about how he just moved into the building, he was new in town and how he didn't know anyone.

As the evaluator doors open, he asked Nikki once again what floor she was going to. He said he didn't mind helping her take her groceries into her apartment. He enjoyed helping people. Nikki had a funny feeling that something wasn't quite right, so she made up the excuse she had to go back to the store to pick up something she forgot.

"That's okay; I can take your groceries up to your apartment and put them away for you while you go back to the store." "Sorry, I don't think my boyfriend would appreciate coming home to a stranger in our apartment while I am out. He will be home shortly, and I need to go back to the store before he arrives home from work." Nikki said as she walked out of the building lobby. Once Nikki felt she was safe, she went to building security to inform them about the incident with the strange man.

The security guard on duty told Nikki that a strange man was going around the neighbourhood trying to get women to let him help them to their apartments. The guard told Nikki that she made the right decision not to let him help her and especially not telling him what floor her apartment was on. The guard took a description of the man from Nikki and escorted her up to her apartment. He said to her that he was going to let the police know of the incident, and will let her know if he hears of any further details.

Know Your Limits

For those of you who enjoy the consumption of adult beverages, do you know your limit? How many drinks can you handle before you lose control of yourself? Knowing your limits is essential to keeping yourself out of potential danger. If you become intoxicated, your judgment becomes impaired. You might end up doing something you normally wouldn't do had you been sober.

Your fine motor skills become impaired, and you don't have the same level of control over your body. If attacked, you won't be able to defend yourself as effectively as when you are sober. You are therefore increasing the chances of you becoming an easier target for an assailant looking for a good time.

If you decide to go beyond your limits, make sure you are with someone like a friend to whom you can trust with your safety and wellbeing. A little precaution ahead of time can go a long way in avoiding potential dangers.

Watch Your Drinks

When you are out at a social gathering or a pub, make sure you keep an eye on your drinks. You don't want to take the chance of someone slipping something into your drink that impairs you physically or mentally. For some reason, you have to leave your drink unattended, best to get yourself a new one instead of taking the risk of drinking a contaminated one. If someone offers to buy or get you a drink, the best practice is to go with them, and get the drink yourself. This way, you know the drink is safe for consumption.

Years ago, one of my cousins and her friends went to a party at a cottage up north on the lake. It was in the middle of summer on a warm night where everyone was drinking, dancing, going for dips in the lake, and having a great time. Good old-fashioned summer fun at the cottage, right?

Well, the next morning, one of the girls woke up on the beach. All of her clothes had been removed and were nowhere to be seen. She had no recollection of what had happened to her from the night before.

No Means No

Whether you have been together for a long time or your relationship is relatively new, when you say no, it means no. It doesn't mean maybe in a few minutes, or slow down a bit. It means to stop because you don't want to go any further.

It is okay for you to start the actions of being intimate with someone and decide you no longer want to continue. You don't have to give a reason for stopping. When you say no or stop, your partner needs to respect your wishes. They should not continue or try to force themselves on you. If they won't stop, you will have to defend yourself until they stop or until you can escape. In this case, you need to report the incident to the authorities.

Sometimes being intoxicated can cloud someone's judgment, and they don't quite understand what they are doing. If you tell them to stop, and they won't, try yelling at them, "Please don't rape me!" Hearing the word rape might snap them out of it. If it doesn't, and they continue, you will have to defend yourself and report the incident to the authorities.

The Statistics show in Canada annually that only 33 sexual assaults are reported out of every 1,000. Out of those 33 reported, 29 are recorded as a crime, 12 have charges laid, 6 are prosecuted, and only 3 lead to a conviction. The statistics show that 997 out of every 1,000 assailants that commit sexual assault get away with it. You must report an incident when it happens. We all need to change these numbers.

One Time Is Too Many

The numbers show that over 50% of women experience physical abuse at least once in their lifetime. The figures also show that over 50% of the offenders are married or in long-term relationships. Basically their husbands or boyfriends are abusing a high percentage of these women.

Most of the time, the abuse happens more than once. It almost becomes a norm in the relationship. But the thing you need to realize is that one time is too many. Once you have been abused one time, it will happen again and again. Once it happens, you need to leave the relationship right away and report the incident. As mentioned earlier, once a week a woman is murdered by her intimate partner, and we don't want that to happen to you.

Don't Be Afraid To Leave

Once a relationship becomes abusive, it is time to leave. For obvious reasons mentioned previously, plus if there are children involved, they need to be removed from the abusive environment. You also need to realize that your abuse is not your fault. The person who is doing the abuse has the problem, not you.

Now, it won't be easy. Most women who find themselves in this position are afraid to leave. Some of their reasons are

- Afraid their partner will come after them and hurt or kill them
- Fearful of surviving on their own financially
- They are worried about what others will think of them
- Believe the abuse will stop
- It is her fault, not his

- Are afraid their abuser will hurt or take away their children

It takes a strong woman to put her fears aside to do what is right for her and her children if she has any. One of the ladies I know was in a very abusive relationship with the father of her child. Before she got pregnant, the relationship wasn't good. They would fight a lot, and sometimes it would get physical with him hitting her. He was also very abusive with his words.

After their child was born, things got worst. One day while the child was at the grandparents for a visit, the mother and father got into another argument. He hit her, knocking her to the ground. He got on top of her and started to strangle her. She told me that she thought she was going to die that day. She felt like she was only a few breaths away from death.

That was the breaking point for her. She kicked him out and spent many years in counselling. She still suffers from the odd episode as a result of all the abuse suffered over the years, especially the final incident. That's what a lot of people don't understand. The trauma can stick with you a long time, even forever.

There's Always Options To Get Help

Once you have decided to leave your abuser, there is help out there for you. On any given night in Canada, over 3,000 women will spend the night in a women's shelter to escape abuse. Almost every community has a women's shelter where you can go for help. A lot of them provide shelter, various programs and counselling, finance help, and so on. A quick Google search will help you find the shelter closes to you.

Other options for help include the local authorities as well as your friends and family. Don't be too proud to reach out for help if you need it. That is what friends and family are for. Remember that you'd do the same for them   too.

CARPOOLING TO WORK

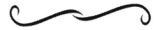

I t's Monday morning, a fresh start to a new workweek. Claire is getting her kids ready for school and making lunches, checking their homework, getting them dressed, etc. The typical start to her workday. Everyone eats breakfast, and out the door they go. The kids hop on the school bus while Claire gets in the car, ready to go pick up Miesha, her work colleague.

Claire drove over to Miesha's house, which is a few blocks away and pulled into her driveway, and waited for Miesha to come out. Miesha and Claire have been working together for a few years at the advertising firm. Miesha came out and put her briefcase in the back of Claire's car, and they drove off.

Their daily commute to work is roughly 30 minutes from Miesha's home, which gives the two ladies a chance to catch up on everything that happened over the weekend. Typical Monday morning chatter. They pulled up to a red light and were waiting for the light to turn green when suddenly the driver's side door open and a hand grabbed Claire's arm.

Without any hesitation, Claire put her foot on the gas pedal and drove forward, causing the hand to let go. She drove around the corner and continued down the street, looking in the rear view mirror to see if she could see if the person who grabbed her was in pursuit. Meanwhile, Miesha was calling 911 to alert the authorities of what just happened to them. One of the things Miesha learned at the self-defense seminar that she and Sally took while in university.

Miesha and Claire have been carpooling for a few years and spent many conversations discussing various situations and what they might do. They have established several plans for different situations that may occur while they are commuting to work or if they are out somewhere together.

CHAPTER SIX
DEALING WITH STRANGERS

You deal with hundreds of strangers every single day. Like we have been saying throughout this book, 99% of people are pretty cool. Most strangers will never trigger your spidey senses and make you feel that there is something wrong. But how do you deal with strangers who make you feel uncomfortable?

You can't assume that every person that makes you feel uncomfortable wants to assault you. That doesn't make any sense and will make you paranoid. However, you should stay alert in case you do run into the one that does. In the meantime, here are some tips to use when dealing with strangers.

Make Friends

This is going to sound a bit odd but make friends with strangers. You are probably thinking, what? I don't mean actually make friends with strangers. Well, you will with some people as that is how you currently have the friends you have now. But that is not what I am talking about. I am referring to being friendly and speaking with people you don't know when out and about.

Especially if there is a stranger nearby that makes you feel uncomfortable and you aren't too sure of. Start up a conversation with someone, so it appears you know him or her. If that stranger was a potential predator, you will most likely deter them from attacking you if they think you are not alone. Don't make it obvious that is what you are trying to accomplish, or they will see right through you.

Refuse With A Smile

One thing I will say that is great about most communities is that there is always someone willing to help out. Most strangers are willing to do little things like holding the door for someone, picking something up that has fallen, paying for the coffee of the person behind them in line, and so on. But there are cases where you should refuse help or an offer, and you do it with a smile because it's hard to get mad at someone who gives you a friendly smile while politely refusing.

If someone offers to do something for you and you can easily do it yourself, and you want to refuse the help, that is okay. Politely refuse with a smile. Most likely, that will end the interaction. If it doesn't stop the interaction and they are being persistent, politely refuse with a smile once again and start talking to someone else or walk away if you need to. In both cases, you would keep an eye on them just to be safe.

When you are out at a social gathering or pub, and someone you don't know offers you a drink, you can politely refuse with a smile. Try saying, "No thanks, I have reached my limits for now, but thanks for thinking of me," while giving a smile. Being polite and acknowledging their generosity at the same time is always a good option.

Talk On The Phone

Most times, I would say talking on the phone in public is a huge distraction. You tend to lose focus on what's happening around you, making you an easier target for a predator looking for their next victim. There are times when talking on the phone can save you though.

When you sense that there is someone who is lurking nearby and is paying a little too much attention to you, your phone can help you. One way is you can call someone on the phone and let that person know what is going on. If the person who is making you uncomfortable is in hearing range, they will realize that you have caught them. There goes their element of surprise. A second way is pretending to call someone if you don't actually want to talk to someone. You should get the same results as the first option, but if something happens to you, no one will know. So make the smart decision for you.

Run Away

One of the best concepts I learned early on in my Martial Arts career was don't be there. More specifically, the best defense you can have is don't be there. So if you find yourself in a situation where you are incredibly uncomfortable, simply walk or run away. There is no need to hang around to find out what might happen. What might happen might not be good for you.

Also, when you find yourself in a situation where you encounter an assailant and physically defending yourself is the only option. Your job is to inflict enough pain and damage that allows you to neutralize the situation and escape by running away. Never stay around to see what will happen. You might find yourself on the receiving end of a brutal attack from someone you now just made extremely angry.

Don't Take Anything From Strangers

There are a lot of friendly people out there who may want to or offer to give you something. It can range from alcoholic drinks, food, coffee, candy, small gifts, and so on. Most times, it is fine to accept these gifts without any risk of harm. But what if it's coming from someone you don't know and it's entirely out of place? You would refuse with a smile like you read about earlier in this chapter. Smiles are powerful.

We teach our children not to take anything from strangers, and the rules apply to us as well. If you run into the wrong person who offers you something, they could be using their offer as a distraction from what they really intend to do to you. They could have done something to a food or drink item that will harm you if you consume it. They also could be using an offering to get you to do something for them, therefore, putting them in control. Proceed with caution and make smart decisions for you.

Arm's Reach From Stranger

When interacting with people that you don't know well or are unsure of, keep them at arm's reach or a little further away. Most people, unless you have a close relationship with them, will naturally maintain a certain distance away. If they impose themselves on you by violating your personal space, they may have ill intent for you. In which case, you should position yourself to maintain an arm's reach distance away or greater from them.

Arm's reach distance away or more reduces the chances of them grabbing or striking you as quickly compared to them being closer to you. Physical space between you and someone else allows you a quicker response time. Not saying you won't get hit or grabbed, but chances of you defending yourself is higher as you will see an attacker sooner.

This also applies when you find yourself in an argument or heated confrontation with someone who decides to throw a punch at you when you are standing right there. You won't have time to react and could get seriously injured or worse.

Talk With Your Hands Up

While maintaining a safe distance, make sure to keep your hands up to help prevent any sort of attack striking you. If someone wants to hit you, they will have to get around your arms somehow. This allows you to respond with the appropriate defenses for that situation with minimum damage done to you in the way of the initial blocks from your arms.

Most people talk with their hands anyway, so it will appear natural for them to be up in front of you. It's not a good idea to be close to someone with your arms crossed, behind your back, or in your pockets. You won't have much of a defense.

You can also use your hands and arms as a physical barrier between you and someone else. If they get too close to you and you can't back away, you can physically put your hands or arms on them. This provides you with a brief moment before you may have to defend yourself with strikes depending on the intent of the other person. We call this technique framing because it creates a frame in which someone has to get around.

Physical Barrier

Sometimes to maintain a safe distance from someone, you have to use a physical barrier between the two of you. A physical barrier can be anything at all that helps prevent someone from touching you.

Some physical barriers could be:

- Car or truck
- A door
- People in a crowd
- Piece of furniture like a chair or table
- Park Bench
- Trees or bushes

A personal example of using physical barriers to keep someone at a safe distance from me happened one night about nine years ago. A few of my adult students and I decided to play billiards at the local pool hall. When we first got there, the place was empty. Great! We have the place all to ourselves. But that wouldn't last long. Shortly after, a group of guys showed up to play billiards as well. All was well, as you would expect until one of the guys said they recognized me and came over.

He was heavily intoxicated, and I will make the strong assumption that he was high on something too. Anyway, he started to get in my space a little, saying he knew who I was. He had been on my Facebook page and was saying something about owing his sister money or something. It was hard to understand him. But you could tell he was looking to pick a fight with me. I had just won the ISKA World Championships, and I was in the newspaper and on the radio. Maybe he wanted to prove himself against a world champion. Who knows?

But he kept trying to get in my space. I kept him a little out of arms reach from me. He was trying everything he could. He would move closer to me, he kept telling me to shake his hand, wanted me to sit with him behind this table because we were friends, and so on. Luckily I was able to use physical space and my words to keep myself safe. But in my head, I was strategizing all the things I could do just in case.

That was a wild night, but luckily I was able to keep my cool and didn't fall for any of his tricks. I still don't understand really what that was all about, and I don't even know his sister, nor do I owe her any money. As an adult, I have never borrowed money from anyone.

Use The Buddy System

Using the buddy system when you are going anywhere where there's going to be a lot of people is something you should consider. Such events as concerts, social gatherings, and sporting events are great for going with someone else. First, it is fun to go with someone else so you can talk and share the experiences. Second, if you encounter a dangerous situation, two heads are always better than one to figure it out and keep each other safe. Third, you are less likely to be approached or attacked when you are in a small group. There is safety in numbers.

Eye Contact

Besides being a polite thing to do, making eye contact with people is an excellent self-defense tool. When you make eye contact with someone, you let him or her know you are paying attention to them and are alert. You can tell a lot about what someone is thinking or when he or she are about to do something based on their eyes.

Paying attention to this will give you the ability to respond faster than if you weren't paying attention to their eyes. You won't be able to respond as well to any sort of physical attack they intend to do, leaving you more vulnerable. Eye contact also shows your confidence, which could deter some potential assailants.

Body Language

Not just with strangers, but also with everyone, reading body language can tell you a lot about what someone's intentions are. There are many ways to read someone's body language for many different purposes. Such purposes can include telling if someone likes you, if someone is lying, if someone lacks confidence. Still, you need to be concerned with the body language that tells you someone intends to hurt you.

Some of the tell signs that someone doesn't have good intentions for you are:

- Clenching their fists

- Invading your personal space

- Lack of eye contact

- Too much eye contact

- Clenching jaw and shoving chin towards you

- Flaring nostrils

- Puffing up the chest

- Dilation of the pupils

- Stepping back into a fighting stance

- Tension in the muscles around the eyes

- Eyebrows lower

- Sudden Movements

- Large Gestures

Paying attention to these signs can allow you to try to diffuse the confrontation or to leave before things get worse. Practitioners of Martial Arts learn to read body language. We can see what our opponents are going to do a bit quicker compared to the average person, which allows us to respond more effectively.

The last fitness kickboxer just left, it was shortly after 9 pm, and I was sorting some papers on my desk. I heard something, so I looked up to see a man standing at the front door. I walked out of my office towards the man and asked him if I could help him. My first thought he wanted information about Taekwondo or Kickboxing, as I came closer to the man, I noticed he was dressed pretty roughly with some cardboard boxes under his one arm. Looking back at the situation, I am going to make an assumption that he was most likely homeless.

The man asked if I had any orange juice. I told him no, I didn't, but he probably could get some at the store right beside the academy. He told me he needed the sugar. So that's when I figured he probably needed some money. So I told him to wait there, and I would grab him some change from the office. As I walked to the office, I kept my eye on him in the mirrors on the walls. As I was walking back towards him with some change in my hand, I saw him reach across his body into his coat.

As he was pulling his hand out, my thoughts were if I see anything that looks like a weapon in his hand, I was going on the defense and attack him before he gets a chance to use it on me. He pulled his hand out, and there was nothing in his hand. He must have been scratching himself or something. I gave him the change; he thanked me and left. I locked the door after him. Thinking afterwards, he must have been diabetic and he needed the sugar because his blood sugar must have been low.

A few takeaways you can gain from this experience. One, you should lock your doors, especially at night, to stop people from coming in unannounced. So I always lock my door right after the last client of the night. Two, you should always be watching what people's hands are doing. You never know when they might attempt to grab, strike, or use a weapon on you. Now, in this case, there was nothing; however, it could have easily been a weapon he was reaching for. Three, have a plan of attack ready in case you need to use it.

What Are Predators Looking For In Potential

Victims

We call them predators because they stalk their potential victims like animals going after their prey in the wild. And just like predators in the wild, these human predators have specific things they look for that can tell them that this potential victim is an easy conquest.

Here is a list of a few things that predators are looking for:

- Victims with broken families or lack of community

- Lack of confidence in how they conduct themselves

- Easy to control and submissive based on body language

- Victim is alone

- People with exaggerated strides, either too short or too long

- Lack of purpose in their steps and body while walking

- Awkward body movements

- Slumped body

- Downward glaze indicating lack of awareness

- Reluctant to make eye contact with people indicating lack of confidence and being submissive

They choose these people as their victims because they are easier to control and isolate. Any signs of strength, defiance, or awareness from the potential target can often be sufficient to cause a predator to look elsewhere for a more suitable cooperative victim. Therefore conveying confidence and awareness can be one of your best defenses, eliminating the potential dangers before they start.

FITNESS KICKBOXING

Miesha put her things in the back seat of Claire's car before hopping into the passenger's seat beside Claire. It was another typical workday started with Claire and Miesha's morning commute to the office. Claire could tell that Miesha had something on her mind this morning. She kept looking at something on her phone between spurts of conversation between the two.

At first, Claire thought maybe it had something to do with Miesha's breakup with her boyfriend a few months back. They both got along well, however Miesha felt something was missing, and it wasn't fair to him to stay together without any real passion in the relationship. So they parted ways as friends. Even though Miesha thought this was the best for both of them, it was still sad.

"Hey, what's on your mind? You seem a little distracted this morning?" asked Claire. "Oh, sorry," replied Miesha. "I was looking at this ad for fitness kickboxing on Facebook. I was thinking of going to check it out tomorrow night. Want to come try it with me?" "Sure, sounds like fun," replied Claire. It's been a while since Miesha did any exercise or running like she used to when she was back in university. Miesha felt that she was at her lowest point in her life athletically.

The next night Claire and Miesha went to the Taekwondo school near where they lived that taught the fitness kickboxing classes. They signed the paperwork in the academy's office so they could try out the kickboxing class. Before their class started, there was an adult Taekwondo class in session. The Taekwondo students were performing powerful blocks, punches, and kicks. Both Miesha and Claire were impressed by the synchronization and power of the students.

The instructor who had his back to Claire and Miesha especially impressed Miesha. He had such a subtle but commanding presence about him. The instructor turned around to show a different angle of the technique he was teaching. It was Logan! The young man she met years ago at the pub but never saw again after he saved her friend Nora from being sexually assaulted.

After the Taekwondo class let out, Master Logan made his way over to where the ladies were standing. "Hey, Miesha, right?" "Yes, I can't believe you remembered me," Miesha replied. "Of course, I did. I knew you'd show up here sooner or later." "Oh, really!" Miesha replied. "Yep, now you better hurry up, class is about to start."

Master Logan put Miesha and Claire through their paces. Various kickboxing combinations on the heavy bags, ground and pound strikes on the mixed Martial Arts body bags, kettlebell swings, and lots of push-ups, to name a few. Oh, and don't forget about the burpees. It was a sweaty workout. Miesha and Claire were both hooked and signed up for classes.

CHAPTER SEVEN
VEHICLE SAFETY

We are commuting to and from work, dropping the kids off at school, picking up groceries, running some errands at the post office, and so on. We spend a lot of time in our cars going to and from various places on any given day. So it makes sense that potential predators might use our vehicle against us. No, I don't mean they will run us over with it, but you never know. That does happen. No, I am talking about attacking you when you are going to and from the car or carjacking you while you are in it.

In this chapter, you will learn various tips and strategies to keep yourself car safe. Learn what you should do when an assailant confronts you, or how to avoid and deter predators from messing with you and your car.

Parked Car

Whenever you park your car, there are a few things that can help you reduce the risk of being surprised by a hidden assailant.

- Park your vehicle away from big trucks or vans where a potential attacker or carjacker can hide behind undetected

- Park your vehicle in such a way that when you are approaching it, you can see the driver side door

- Park your car in a well-lit area or under a light so you can see everything around it and you will be seen if something were to happen

- Park somewhere where you can remember where the car is, so you don't go wandering around looking for it

- Lock your doors at all times

Carjacking While Parked

Carjackers generally look for one of two things happening. One, they are watching you as you approach your vehicle, and they will try to catch you off guard. Generally, after you already have the keys in the door of the car. You are making it easier for them to get in without messing around with the keys themselves. Two, you are exiting the vehicle, and they attack while the door is still open. In both scenarios, you are, in most cases, distracted by the actions you are taking to get in or out of the vehicle and not paying attention to anything else.

In cases where a carjacker wants to steal your car and nothing else, and there are no children with you, play it safe and let them take it. Your life is more valuable than the vehicle. However, in cases where you have children with you, you will need to respond quickly and take care of the assailant. You should discuss with children about what to do if a carjacking happens to you. Discuss what you will do and what they should do. Your primary actions will be to keep the children safe, and their first actions will be to get away as fast as possible.

When Approaching Your Car

When approaching your vehicle, whether it's in a parking lot at the mall, bank, work, or at home, you should be actively looking around to make sure it is safe. Look around to see who and what is in the immediate area. You want your keys in your hand and ready to unlock the door if your vehicle requires that. A lot of newer vehicles you can have your keys in your pocket, and the car will open for you. Either way, be ready to open your door when you get to your vehicle. Don't fumble around with the keys at your car. You leave yourself open for an attack or carjacking.

When you are carrying something to your car, make sure it is well organized and easy to manage. If you are struggling with what you are carrying, this opens you up for an attack because you are not focusing on being alert. Plus, you won't be able to defend yourself, as your hands will be tied up with what you are trying to manage. If at all possible, carry your belongings in one arm while holding your keys in the other hand.

When putting things away or getting the children in the car, make sure you are actively looking around so that no one can sneak up on you. When alone, don't take too much time to put stuff in the car or take off. The longer you sit around, the higher the chances someone can catch you off guard. Also, when sitting in your car, make sure the windows are up, and the doors are locked so no one can reach in or open the door to grab you.

Someone is Approaching

If someone is approaching you while you are outside of your car and you feel threatened, you should acknowledge their presence. Tell them to back off if needed. Get in your vehicle and lock the door if you are able too. When in the car, sound the horn to cause attention to your assailant. The loud noise should cause them to leave in a hurry. If they are still approaching, be prepared to drive away. They are responsible for their own safety. i.e., I am not telling you to run them over.

If you weren't able to get in the car, run away if possible while causing a scene to draw attention to the assailant. If you are not able to escape, remember your strengths and their weaknesses. Do what you have to do to keep yourself safe and escape as soon as you can. Report the incident as soon as you can.

Exiting Your Car

When exiting your vehicle, you want to take the same amount of care as you do approaching and getting into your car. Before shutting off the ignition or unlocking the door, take a moment to look around to see who and what is in your immediate area. If everything looks good and it is safe to do so, exit the vehicle and lock the door and go to where you are heading. Be alert for anyone in the area or if someone is following you. The same protocol applies here as the previous paragraph if someone is approaching you or following you.

Car Safety While Driving

All kinds of things can happen while driving. Trust me, I've seen enough of it while both being the driver and being the passenger—so many things to look out for when trying to drive and stay safe at the same time. Here is a list of things to keep in mind:

- Watch out for other people's bad driving

- Keep your doors locked and windows up while driving and stopping for traffic lights

- If you have children in the car, know where each one is seated

- Don't keep valuable items in the car

- Avoid parking near big vans or trucks that you cannot see around

- Always have a cell phone handy

- Plan out your routes ahead of time

- Avoid heavy traffic if possible

- Have plans of action if emergencies happen

- Make sure your passengers know your emergency action plans

- Keep your vehicle well maintained so less likelihood of something going wrong

- Don't go with a stranger if you run out of gas, have them bring some gas back in a container

- Fill up your vehicle with gas regularly to reduce the risk of running out of fuel

Implementing these guidelines will help reduce the risks of something terrible happening to you. Preparing for the worse helps prevents the worse from happening.

Carjacking While Driving

Carjacking doesn't just happen while you are parked. It can happen while the engine is on and you are sitting at the stoplight waiting for it to turn green. Another vehicle can easily pull up beside you, and an assailant can jump out and open your car door just like that. So number one, keep your doors locked at all times. In a lot of modern cars the doors lock themselves when the vehicle is in gear. But in case they don't, you should double-check the doors are locked.

In a case where the door is opened, and someone grabs your arm, if there is no one in front of you and you can safely do so, drive forward. Your assailant should let go, and in most cases, they won't try a second attempt. Too dangerous and the risk of getting caught is now much higher. Always take this option if you have children in the car. Their safety is your number one priority, even if you have to drive up on the sidewalk to escape the carjacker. If you are by yourself and can't drive away due to heavy traffic or something, you may have to let your carjacker have your vehicle. Remember, your life is more valuable than your car.

Averil was working late at the office, which is a regular occurrence. She is always working well after everyone else leaves. Averil collected her belongings and rode the elevator to the building's underground parking lot. She got out and headed in the general direction of where she parked her car.

As per most parking garages at night, it was dark and eerie due to poor lighting. The odd light bulb was flickering, making it hard to see in some sections of the parking garage. Averil always felt uneasy walking from the elevator to her car so she would hurry in her steps.

She often wondered if staying late after everyone else has gone was worth the effort.

Averil put her purse and belongings on the trunk lid of her car while she rummaged through her coat pockets for her keys. As she was searching for her keys, they fell out of her pocket and landed under her car. She got down on her hands and knees, reaching under the car, hoping to find them, feeling around for what felt like forever before finding them.

She stood up, opened her trunk with the keys, and placed her belongings in. She closed the trunk lid, went around the car to the driver's side door. She was putting the keys in the lock when suddenly Averil felt something shoved in her back. "Don't scream or turn around, or I will shoot." said a deep voice. Averil, frozen in fear, stood there with tears starting to build up in her eyes, unable to speak.

"I want you to close your eyes, place your hands on the back of your head and take a few steps back from the car." calmly said her carjacker. "Now, get on your knees, don't open your eyes or move until I am gone." Averil did as commanded. She listened as the car door slammed shut, the engine fired up, and the car drove away. Averil remained still keeping her eyes closed until her car was no longer audible in the now quiet parking garage. She remained still for a few extra moments, afraid her carjacker was still lurking nearby.

Are You Being Followed?

While driving, you should be checking in your mirrors to see if anyone looks suspicious or is following you. Predators will follow you for multiple reasons such as you have something they want, they want to scare you, they want your car, or perhaps they even want you. Things can get really scary when another vehicle is following you. Who knows what their intentions are for you.

The first thing you need to do is be alert, practicing your situational awareness skills, and using the five-second rule continuously. Some ways to figure out if someone is following you are, they keep changing directions or lanes when you do, they adjust their vehicle speed when you do, and they keep showing up everywhere you go. This also applies if you are walking as well, not just driving in your vehicle.

If you believe that you are being followed, you can pull into a nearby gas station and ask the attendant for help. You can drive to the closest police station or fire department if you know where they are located. Call the police on your cell phone and tell them what is going on. They will give you directions to follow. If possible, don't drive to your home, or a friend's or family member's home either. You will be letting the person who is following you know where you live or where someone you care about lives. No matter what you decide to do, don't try to confront the person who has been following you. You don't know what their intentions are.

Road Rage

Road rage is a serious problem that has cost many innocent people their lives. The best thing to do is stay calm while driving and ignore anyone else who is being rude or otherwise. If you feel you are being a victim of someone's road rage, pull off somewhere safe and call the authorities or get help. Don't confront the person or get out of your vehicle—the same protocols apply as with dealing with carjackers.

11pm could not come any faster most nights. This time of night, it always seems that the questionable people started to lurk around. They were doing their business when most of the world was asleep. Activities that are not entirely legitimate.

Emma is a 30ish single mom who works late nights cleaning offices to make ends meet to support her two young children. She is lucky that her parents pitch in to help her by watching Emma's children while she does her cleaning jobs after hours. Her parents often worried that something terrible was going to happen to Emma because she was alone at these offices late at night. Emma would always reassure her parents that the doors are locked, and no one could get in. Emma's parents were more worried about her walking to her car alone. Anything could happen at that time of night.

One of Emma's cleaning clients is a dentist office located in one of the rougher areas of the city. One night as Emma was locking up, she noticed a strange car parked on the street near the dentist office that is usually not there. For a few nights in a row, the car just sat in the same spot. Then a few nights after Emma noticed the car now parking at the far end of the parking lot belong to the dentist office. The windows of the car are heavily tinted, so Emma could not see if anyone was in the car.

About a week went by with the car parking at the far end of the parking lot; now it was moving closer each night. Emma was starting to get quite nervous about locking up at the end of her shift and going to her car. It was now the end of the week, and Emma was locking up when the car drove into the parking lot and was heading towards Emma. She unlocked the door and went back into the building and locked the door behind her. The car just sat in front of the door with the headlights shining towards the dentist office.

After a while, the car parked at the end of the parking lot, waiting for Emma to come out. Once she noticed the car was across the lot, Emma decided she could run for her car safely. So Emma quickly locked the door and ran for her car. She wasted no time starting the car and driving out of the parking lot. The strange vehicle followed her out of the parking lot.

The car followed Emma across town, keeping at a distance so she wouldn't notice the car was following her. Emma pulled into her parents' driveway, and while getting out of her car; the other car slowly drove by. A distraught Emma ran into her parents' house and called the police. When the police arrived, she told them what had just happened and about the past few weeks. The police figured they were trying to get Emma's keys for the dentist office because of the drugs inside. They also told Emma that they would be monitoring the building for the suspicious car. If this were to happen again, Emma was to stay where she was and call the police right away. Emma was lucky that nothing serious happened to her.

Car safety is the same as any other area of personal safety. Practice good situational awareness and have plans for various situations so you can respond quickly with the best and safest options for you. Also, discuss your vehicle safety plans with anyone who drives with you, so they know what to do if something happens. When something happens, little communication occurs between you and your passengers. Everyone needs to know what to do to ensure the safety of everyone else without much thought.

A FUTURE BLACK BELT

Miesha and Claire have been attending their fitness kickboxing classes for about six months now. Both ladies have lost some unwanted body fat, toned up their muscles, and have gotten a lot stronger. The workouts are tough, but Miesha loves them. She especially loved the kicking on the heavy bags. Some of the other ladies would stop and watch when Miesha was kicking on the bags. Wham! The impact of her roundhouse kicks!

During the workout one evening, Miesha was working over one of the heavy bags with her jab-cross roundhouse kick combination while Master Logan was watching. "You have great kicks," Master Logan said to Miesha. "Really?" "Yeah, you should consider trying Taekwondo class. I think you will really like it." "Okay, I will give it a try. Thank you," replied Miesha.

Miesha's next class, she got her Taekwondo dobuk, Korean for uniform, and waited for the children's class to finish up. She was a bit nervous about going into a group where everyone else knew what they were doing. Master Logan bowed out the children's class and went over to the back of the dojang where Miesha was waiting. "Ready to go?" "Yep, sure am'" replied Miesha. "Good, don't be nervous, you have wicked kicks. You will do great," Master Logan encouraged Miesha.

During her first Taekwondo class, Miesha trained various punches, blocks, forms, self-defense techniques, and her favourite, kicking, of course. It was a great workout with an emphasis on learning how to protect yourself from various attacks someone might encounter. Miesha was hooked. There was a sense of empowerment that drew her in.

"Well?" Master Logan asked. "Yep, I really enjoyed it. Can't wait for the next class," Miesha replied. "I knew you'd love it. You're going to make a great Black Belt someday," Master Logan had a feeling that Miesha was going to go far in Martial Arts. He could feel it.

CHAPTER EIGHT
TRAVELLING AND VACATIONS

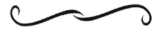

Travelling and vacations is going to be a smaller chapter as most of the tips and strategies that we have already discussed also apply when you are on vacation. We will touch on a few things that you have previously seen and go over a few things you may not have considered yet.

Be Alert While on Vacation

Situational awareness is just as critical on vacation as it is in your daily routines—new surroundings with new people and new cultures to experience. You will most likely be a little distracted with all these new experiences, which makes tourists like you an easier target for the local predators. They can always spot a tourist. They seem out of place and sometimes clueless. Always be alert.

Don't Look Like A Tourist

One of the things you have to try to avoid is looking like a tourist. You want to blend in with the locals, so you are less likely to fall prey to a local criminal. Be alert of your surroundings and learn the customs of the area you will be visiting ahead of time. The more you know about the area you are going to, the more you can fit in.

Be On The Watch Out For Scams

In certain parts of the world the locals prey on the tourists. They scam them with fake products and tours. Make sure you only go to legitimate stores and businesses to purchase merchandise to prevent getting ripped off. Only go on tours provided by the resorts or legitimate tour companies. There are a lot of fake tours out there that rip off the tourists. Some fake tours are a cover up for robbing the tourists when they get them isolated and alone.

Bribes

In some places around the world, the authorities are used to bribes and payoffs to help compensate for their low income. Be prepared to be paying them for entering the country, travelling to specific locations, and leaving the country. If you don't pay them, you can expect to end up in jail. So be ready with some extra cash on hand.

Checking In When Travelling

When travelling, especially alone, you should be checking in with someone back home. Let that person know you have arrived at your location safely. While on vacation, you should be checking in periodically with that person. If they haven't heard from you in a predetermined time, they have permission to reach out to you, and if you don't reply, they can initiate a process to find you.

Don't Let Anyone Know You Are Alone

When travelling alone, don't let anyone know you are alone. If a potential predator knows you are alone on vacation, they might try to take advantage of you. Never provide your personal details to anyone.

Don't Let Strangers In Your Hotel Room

Just like your home, don't let strangers come into your hotel room. You don't know their intent, and if they have bad intentions for you, you won't have anywhere to escape to. Plus, never let strangers know where your hotel room is. There is a reason why hotel staff won't tell you which room another person is staying in.

Stay In Safe Hotels

There are plenty of hotels to stay at when travelling. Make sure you do your research ahead of time and stay at hotels that are reputable and in safe locations. Questionable locations will bring suspicious guests with questionable activities.

Backup Copies Of Government Issued Documents

Make backup copies of all your government issued documents when you are travelling—such documents as driver's license, health card, passport, and birth certificate. Keep your originals on you and a copy of them in the safe in your hotel room. If you lose your documents, you have a backup copy to prove your identity.

Cash Versus Credit and Bank Cards

When travelling, you need to decide if you are going to use cash, travel cheques, bankcard, or credit cards. Or are you going to be using a mixture of them all? Whatever you decide, never take your eyes off your bank or credit cards. You don't want anyone stealing your cards information or your identity.

Know Your Travel Plans

Plan out your travels. Know how you are going to get there, and how are you going to get back. What methods of transportation are you taking? Where are you staying? That's the purpose of your trip? What are all the things you will need to know? The more you plan, the safer you can be. You tend to save a lot more money with a well planned out trip too.

The sun was shining, the tropical birds were singing, and you could smell the fresh saltwater in the air. It's a great way to wake up on your first day on the islands, Zoey thought. Zoey arrived at the resort late last night and went right to bed, not seeing any of the beauty where she would be spending her vacation alone. She needed the much-deserved time off from work and life in general. She was always busy and never really took any time to enjoy herself.

Zoey was looking forward to reading on the beach, swimming in the ocean, hanging out poolside, enjoying all the different foods of the locals, and of course, the tours around the islands. There was plenty for her to do. The challenge was where she should start. Relaxing isn't one of Zoey's strong points as she is always on the go. After unpacking her bags and putting everything away, she decided she would start with breakfast at one of the beachside restaurants at the resort.

Breakfast was delicious and made Zoey's morning. Next, Zoey decided to go on one of the many guided tours offered by the resort. She went over to the bus area where the various guided tours departed from the resort. Zoey chose the day tour that she wanted to go on and jumped on the bus. The bus took them all over the island, showing them all the typical tourist attractions. The tour guide was excellent at describing the history of each location that they visited. After a long day of touring, the bus took the tourists back to the resort. While everyone was getting off the bus, the tour guide mentioned to everyone that no one should go out exploring without one of the tour guides from the resort.

The next day Zoey started her day by reading on the beach and soaking up some sun. It's been a while since she had a bikini on in public probably since she was in college, which was a good fifteen years ago. Zoey was in great physical shape as she usually workouts every morning to start her day on the right foot. While reading her book, a handsome young man came along and sat beside Zoey.

"You're not from around here, are you?" the young man said to Zoey. "No, I am actually on vacation," Zoey replied. "I thought so." "and how could you tell?" she replied. "I can always pick out the tourists to the islands. Which resort are you staying at?" the man asked. "I am staying right over there," Zoey replied, pointing to the resort to their right. "I got in two nights ago." "Excellence, what did you get up to yesterday?" "I went on a guided tour provided by the resort." "How was that?" asked the man. "It was okay," Zoey replied, "They took us to all the typical tourist attractions."

"Well, how would you like to see some of the sights only locals to the island know about?" "That would be great, but we just met, and I don't even know your name," replied Zoey. "Jack's the name, and what's yours?" "Zoey" "Zoey, what a beautiful name for a beautiful woman. Now that we aren't strangers anymore, how about that personally guided tour?" Blushing, Zoey agreed. Jack and Zoey went back to Zoey's resort so she could change and get ready.

Jack took Zoey to the various sights all over the island that only the locals knew existed. Near the end of the day, Jack and Zoey went to this one seaside cliff overlooking the ocean as the sun was setting. If one didn't know better, you would swear you were looking at a small piece of heaven. Zoey was in awe when Jack reached into his pocket and pulled out a knife. "Give me all the cash you have on you," Jack demanded as he pointed the knife at Zoey. After giving Jack all the cash she had on her, Jack told her not to tell any one, as he knew what room she was staying in at the resort. With that, Jack left Zoey all alone at the seaside cliff.

You are far more vulnerable while on vacation and travelling than you are when you are at home in your local community. Your situational awareness skills have to be on high alert. Like we discussed before, 99% of strangers are pretty cool, but there still is the 1% that aren't. These are the ones you have to watch out for because you won't have the same support team while abroad.

BLACK BELT TESTING

How did I get myself to this point Miesha was thinking to herself as she walked towards Master Logan. It was only yesterday that she spent 10 hours with a bunch of her fellow Taekwondo students being pushed to their limits and beyond. Now she was walking across the stage towards her Taekwondo Master, holding her Black Belt in his hands.

The Black Belt candidates were filing into the dojang and prepping all their equipment and food for the day. It was going to be a long ten hours of Black Belt testing. The test would cover everything that the Black Belt candidates have learned so far in their Martial Arts careers. Miesha was confident that she knew everything she had to know but was nervous about the uncertainty of how the day would unfold.

The test started with the Masters and Instructors explaining the rules of the testing and words of encouragement to help get the candidates through the day. First up was the hour-long warm up/fitness portion to test the physical and mental endurance of the candidates. After everyone was good and sweaty, they moved on to the basics portion. Going over various punches, strikes, blocks, defenses, and stances.

Moving along, they were tested on their traditional forms. Traditional forms are routines of various blocks, strikes, kicks, and stances put into self-defense sequences performed by ones' self in solo practice. Once done their forms, they moved into kicking—one of Miesha's favourite parts of Taekwondo besides self-defense. The candidates worked single kicks, two and three kick combos, and finished with some endurance kicking leaving them exhausted. Still, the day wasn't over with yet.

Miesha was standing across the ring, staring at her opponent for this sparring match. Sparring was not one of her favourite parts of Taekwondo but knew it was essential to practice. Sparring helps the practitioner work on reaction and response timing, distancing, strategy, physical conditioning, and control. Not just the physical control of her techniques, but control of her emotional responses to someone trying to hit or score a point on her in a controlled environment of sparring.

Miesha and her opponent were called to the center of the ring. They bowed to each other and got into their fighting stances. The referee dropped his hand, signalling the start of the match. The two Black Belt candidates started circling each other. Miesha was paying close attention to the slightest of movements her opponent was making that would tell Miesha what was about to happen. Her opponent fired off the opening kick. The two went back and forth exchanging punching and kicking combinations trying to one-up each other. Finally, what seemed like forever, the referee called for the stop of the match. The time had expired.

The candidates were then tested on their one-step sparring and self-defense requirements. First, demonstrating the various techniques to show they knew them before performing live attack drills to simulate the chaotic nature of self-defense scenarios in the real world. Finally, the last requirement the candidates had to complete during the testing was board breaking. Breaking is a test of ones' power, strength, and skill against material that appears harder than your own body.

Miesha broke her one-inch pine boards with a punch, an elbow strike, snap kick, and a 360-degree roundhouse kick. Her last break was a power elbow strike on a stack of multiple boards blasting through them like they weren't even there.

The Black Belt was wrapped around Miesha's waist, and the knot was tied. Miesha looked down at her new Black Belt with her name in golden lettering both in English and Korean. It was now real. She is now a Black Belt in Taekwondo after four years of hard training. Lots of tough times, but all the challenges she had faced were worth this one moment in time. She was standing on stage with her Master and fellow Taekwondo Black Belts.

CHAPTER NINE
DAY-TO-DAY HABITS

D ecided to call this chapter "Day-To-Day" because it contains a little of everything that is not in previous chapters but is a part of your day to day. Just a few little habits can add up to how safe you are during your day. So let's take a look at home safety first.

Home Safety

Just because you are at home doesn't mean you are 100% safe. It would be nice if we lived in a world where it was, but unfortunately, we don't. A lot of crimes and assaults actually happen within the home. In fact, 80% of all sexual assaults occur in the home. So you must practice good safety habits each day while at home.

First, you can make sure that you lock your doors and windows, whether at home or not. Now I am not saying you have to lock your house up like a bank vault when you are home, just make sure unwanted visitors can't just come in at will. When the weather is nice out and you want to let some fresh air in, be sure to keep the screen door locked. It applies for windows too. Also, you should keep everything locked up when it's dark out. Predators are more likely to enter your home under cover of night when no one can see them.

Second, when home alone, make sure you are careful whom you let in your home. You should avoid letting random strangers in your home. You never know what their intentions could be. Now there are always exceptions to the rules. If you need to let the plumber in or a cable repair guy in, that is different. But you should be cautious and alert while they are in your home as well. Better to be prepared and have a plan than be assaulted or robbed.

Third, if someone has entered your home unannounced, do you have an escape plan? One of the scariest things you can experience is that of someone breaking into your home while you are home alone and you don't know where they are. If you can lock yourself into a room where the assailant cannot get you, do that first if you cannot escape. Then while in the locked room, call 911 and let them know what is going on. If you can escape by getting outside safely, do so as soon as you can and run to a neighbour's house. Call 911 from there.

If you have children in the house, you need to get them out of the house as fast as you can and only if you can do so safely. If there is no safe way to get them out of the house, lock them and you into a room where the assailant can't get the children or you and call 911. In either case where you are alone or with children and you cannot escape, and you cannot get to a phone, signal the neighbours by turning the lights off and on signalling to them something is wrong. Alternatively, open and shut the blinds to get someone's attention.

Fourth, you should pay attention to the local traffic, both vehicles and foot traffic for suspicious activity. Living in a given spot for a while, you will get to know the cars and foot traffic from the neighbours. If you are practicing good awareness, you will notice suspicious activity from people who don't belong in your community. It's essential to pay attention to cars driving by or people walking by that you didn't notice before. Are they stalking you or a neighbour? Are they scouting the area for a potential robbery? Pay attention to these activities.

Cell Phone Safety

Everyone is glued to his or her cell phones nowadays, an escape from the everyday world and distracted from your surroundings. Whether you are looking at the screen, listening to music, or talking to someone, they take up a lot of your attention. When in public, try to use your phone less and be more engaged with your surroundings and the people that are around you. If you have to use your phone while in public, make sure you are practicing your situational awareness. Predators will look for potential victims that are distracted, like a person on the phone.

Cyber Safety

We are living in the Internet age, with so much information and entertainment at our fingertips. You can access almost anything or anyone with relative ease, which is the scary thing. With virtually everyone on social media or with their address and telephone number listed on various websites, you can look up or find anyone you want. Which means predators have access to your information too.

To help combat this, there are a few simple things you can practice on the Internet:

- Limit your personal information you share on your social media accounts like your home address, work address, email address, and telephone numbers

- Watch out for who you are interacting with online

- Don't give anyone you don't know too much personal information online

- Make your telephone number unlisted so it won't show up in online searches or in the phone books

- Watch out for catfish on dating sites and social media (Catfish are people who take on fake identities to deceive others online, typically in a romantic scenario to gain control of financials or to compromise their victim into doing something)

- Watch out what you post online because once you post it, it never completely goes away

- Avoid arguments and confrontations online

- If you have children, watch out what they are doing online

- Block anyone you don't want to interact with online and block them from seeing your social media accounts

- Report anyone to the social media companies of suspicious or unwanted interactions with someone you have blocked

- Contact authorities if you feel any online interactions could be a physical threat to you

Being alert online is the same as being alert in your day-to-day interactions. Pay attention to everything that is going on, and don't get caught up with all the distractions. Predators will sneak up on you while you are distracted. Staying alert online is staying safe online.

Organize Your Belongings That You Carry

Fumbling around with your belongings makes you a potential victim to a predator who is lurking by. They see that you are distracted and not aware of your surroundings. This allows them to catch you off guard. Having your belongings well organized will enable you to be more alert and engaged with your surroundings while you're going about your day.

It was a sweltering evening in the middle of July. The air conditioning was not working once again. The A/C repair guy came earlier in the day but wasn't able to get it working. Paulie had the fans on, and all the doors and windows open, hoping to cool the house down a bit. Her sports bra and shorts were clinging to her body soaked in sweat. Her husband was away on a business trip, so she was left to look after the house herself.

Paulie thought she would try to cool off by taking a cold shower. The cold water felt so good and refreshing, just what Paulie needed on such a hot night. She was wandering around the kitchen, drying off her hair when she thought she heard a noise coming from the back room. She stopped to listen but heard nothing more. So Paulie shrugged it off, figuring it was the cat.

A few moments later, she heard the noise again. So Paulie went to investigate what the sound was. She walked in the back room, looking around to see what was causing the noise. With a towel wrapped around her body and the towel she used on her hair in her hand. Suddenly the cat jumped out from behind the couch, startling Paulie, causing her to drop her towel.

She bent over to pick up her towel and turned around to walk out of the room when suddenly she was face to face with a man standing in the doorway. He suddenly lunged forward and covered her mouth with his hand preventing her from screaming. He pinned her to the floor and started to remove Paulie's towel. She managed to get her legs up and put her feet on his hips and pushed the man away. As he went to pull himself closer to Paulie, she started kicking him in the face, breaking his nose. As he jerked back, grabbing his nose in pain, Paulie got up and ran out of the room and out the back door.

Paulie ran over to the neighbor's and banged on their door. The couple living came to the door to the sight of Paulie standing on their front porch in nothing but a towel. She told them what just happened and they called 911 for Paulie. The police, fire rescue, and ambulance showed up a few moments later. After investigating, the police informed Paulie that her assailant came in through the back door but there were no signs of forced entry. Paul said she had all the doors open to let the air in because the A/C was not working. The police figured the man must have entered Paulie's house while she was in the shower.

Your day-to-day habits will play a significant role in your safety. It will decrease the chances of you being involved in a situation you don't want to be in. Now you can't control what every person does out there, but you can certainly control what you do. Practice good safety habits both in and out of the home.

WOMEN'S EMPOWERMENT

Sally was sitting in her car, watching a bunch of ladies go into the Taekwondo academy where the women's empowerment and self-defense workshop was taking place. It had been several years since the night her fiancée slapped her across the face. That was the night she had enough. He went to hit her a second time when Sally blocked his arm, grabbing hold of his shoulders and kneeing him in the groin a few times before elbowing him in the face breaking his jaw. "I don't deserve to be treated this way. Now get the hell out before I call the police,' she screamed, tears running down her cheeks.

Miesha and Master Logan were going over the notes for the empowerment workshop and discussing little details while the attendees were making their way into the academy. Miesha happened to glance over at the entranceway of the dojang and saw Sally standing there. The two hadn't seen each other since that night at the restaurant. "Excuse me for a second; I have to go say hi to an old friend." "Yeah sure," Master Logan replied, holding Miesha's notes for her.

"Hey, long time no see." "I know, and I am sorry," replied Sally. "No need to be sorry. It's nice to see you. How's everything going?" "Everything's good. I broke up with my fiancée the night you and I were at the restaurant, and I met someone new a few years back." Sally continued to tell Miesha everything that happened that night, and about all the physical abuse before the night he hit her. She was ashamed, and that is why she didn't tell Miesha before. Sally now had the strength to see her friend Miesha again, and to take part in the workshop Miesha and Master Logan were teaching together.

Miesha and Master Logan started the empowerment workshop with a fifteen-minute discussion on essential concepts and strategies that every woman should to know about self-defense to help keep themselves safe as well as their families and friends. Such concepts included the five-second rule, trusting your intuition, looking and acting confident, know your strengths, vehicle smarts, and a few other important ones. These concepts would continuously come up throughout the workshop, as the various concepts directly relate to specific self-defense techniques and scenarios

Demonstrating the self-defense techniques on Master Logan was one of Miesha's favourite parts of teaching these workshops. Besides inspiring and empowering women with the knowledge to protect themselves, she could be pretty rough on him to show how effective the techniques can be without fear of hurting him. Plus, the attendees seemed to enjoy it, so it added some comedy to the mix, lightening up the mood of a sensitive but essential subject.

After the empowerment workshop was over, Miesha introduced Sally to Master Logan. "Nice to meet you, Sally. Miesha has told me a lot about you." "You too. You and Miesha run a great self-defense workshop. Very inspiring and empowering for the women," Sally said. "Thanks, but I am just the guy who gets beat up by Miesha," laughed Master Logan. "I don't beat you up..." Miesha said as she kicks him in the ribs while giving him the look. "See what I mean," Master Logan said to Sally while laughing. "Truthfully, Miesha, and you really inspired me today. What do I need to do to start Taekwondo classes?"

CHAPTER TEN
REPORTING INCIDENTS

In your lifetime, an incident will either happen to you or someone else you know. Unfortunately, there's 100% likelihood that this will be true. If not to you, then to someone you know, and you will be there when it's happening, or you will find out about it shortly after.

When an incident occurs, someone should report it to the local authorities, such as the police. There are a few main reasons why. One, the police can find and arrest the assailant, which could help prevent the assailant from committing the crime against someone else. Two, it helps prevent the incident from happening to you again. Three, the more the authorities know the numbers and types of incidents happening, the better they can adjust their resources to help prevent and deal with specific types of events and crimes.

Unfortunately, a large number of incidents don't get reported. For example, roughly 460,000 sexual assaults happen in Canada every year. For every 1,000 assaults, only 33 incidents are reported to the police. 29 of these 33 are reported as a crime—twelve incidents where charges are laid. Six are prosecuted, and only three are convicted. Nine hundred ninety-seven assailants walk away free.

Looking at the numbers above, you can agree with me that there needs to be something done. One of them is reporting all incidents. If predators know they can get away with it, they will continue to assault women because there are no consequences for them. Such a horrific reality we live in.

But why are there such a high number of sexual assault incidents not being reported? There are a few reasons we will touch upon here. One of the biggest reasons is the victim feel ashamed. They don't want to tell anyone as they are afraid people will think less of them, or it's their fault. Not a rational thought but their thoughts nonetheless. Two, they are so scared that their assailant might harm them or worse if they report them. As you saw in the numbers in previous paragraphs, most assailants who are reported walk free, leaving them able to go after their accuser/victim or their friends and family.

Three, they are afraid that no one will believe them. It is the victim's word again their assailant. Will the authorities or anyone else believe them? Most victims don't think anyone will believe them. Then if no one believes them, now the accused assailant might go after them.

One way you and I can start to help make things better when it comes to the number of sexual assaults happening is to convince all victims regardless of their fears to report to the police. There is strength in numbers, and if you and I can somehow empower the victims to stand up to their assailants together, we can start to make some progress. Not sure how we can do this, but it is worth some thought and effort.

Even though we mainly focused on sexual assaults and incidents of that nature, all crimes and incidents need to be reported regardless. The police and authorities need to know what the real numbers are so they can better learn how to allocate their resources. The more incidents that are reported with more convictions coming, as a result, should help deter future crimes over a more extended period of time.

Now touching on one of the fears from earlier, if you report a sexual assault or any other crime to the police and they don't believe you, or they just brush it off, speak to another police officer. Like in any other profession out there, there are good police officers who do their jobs well and others that don't. Let's not focus on poor ones but rather the good ones. They will help you. I have personally seen where one officer brushed off an incident as "fine" while the next officer had an issue with the incident and looked into it.

So don't take no for an answer. Stand up for your rights to be heard. Report any incident you become involved with regardless of your fears. You've got to be strong. That's the only way you can fight back against predators. It is also your responsibility to convince anyone who you find out has been a victim but hasn't reported the incident to do so. Neither you nor they can allow the assailant to get away with their crimes. There is too much at stake otherwise.

CLOSING TO EMPOWERED

Now that you have read this book from cover to cover and you have a good grasp on the fundamental concepts and strategies that will help increase the chances of keeping you safe, you now need to go back and review anything you may have missed during the first reading. The more often you take this book out and read it, the more you will engrave these concepts into your daily routines. It's no different than learning a new skill. It takes hundreds of repetitions before you start getting good at it. Implementing the strategies within these pages is no different.

As you saw throughout the book, most of these concepts and strategies intertwine with each other. It's hard for one to exist without another one showing the complexity of any given scenario that could occur. No two situations will be exactly the same. So relying on a few select concepts and ignoring the rest can be dangerous. You must be familiar with as many of these strategies and ideas as you can and continue to add new ones. You must also be actively using them daily. Over time they will become second nature to you so you won't have to think about all of them all the time actively. Doing this will make self-protection as natural as breathing.

I hope you found the information and stories within the pages of *Empowered: Essential Concepts and Strategies Every Woman Should Know About Self-Defense* extremely valuable. If you enjoyed this book, please consider recommending it to all your friends and leave an honest review on Amazon. Your support is greatly appreciated, and I want to say Thank You and wish you all the best in your journey of self-empowerment and defense.

Manufactured by Amazon.ca
Bolton, ON